TEA CLEANSE

Lose Weight, Improve Health, Detox & Reset Your Metabolism

(The Best Tea Detox Recipes for Health and Wellness)

Margie Jackson

I0092615

Published by Sharon Lohan

© Margie Jackson

Tea Cleanse: Lose Weight, Improve Health, Detox & Reset Your Metabolism (The Best Tea Detox Recipes for Health and Wellness)

ISBN 978-1-990334-39-9

Legal & Disclaimer

The information contained in this book is not designed to replace or take the place of any form of medicine or professional medical advice. The information in this book has been provided for educational and entertainment purposes only.

Table of contents

Part 1

1

Introduction

Most of us are constantly worried about our sudden weight gain. What's even worse than gaining weight is the fact that we can't shed it. We are invariably on the hunt for the perfect detox diet that can help us get rid of all the toxins. A tea cleanse diet is the ideal solution to all your weight worries and upset tummies. In this book, we are providing you proven tea cleanse diet strategies that can give you the perfect results.

The diet program mentioned in the book has been well researched and is guaranteed to leave you feeling a few pounds lighter. However, you may not experience drastic weight loss results. You will be able to lose weight gradually by following this diet plan, but the results are sure to last for a longer period. Tea cleanse diet will help you find the new you while giving you the desired weight loss results.

We have also put together tea cleanse recipes to make your weight loss journey easier. While you can feel free to tweak the recipes occasionally, ensure that you stay away from refined sugar and all sorts of fizzy drinks. The diet program in this book is carefully designed to get you that much needed kick-start to detoxification that you have been looking.

So, get ready to revamp your wardrobe because soon you are going to need pants that are few inches smaller. What are we waiting for? Let's get started. Happy reading.

Chapter 1: what is the tea cleanse diet?

How often do you feel tired, have sleepless nights or feel that you have gained weight that you are unable to shed off? Unfortunately, a lot of us are responsible for the havoc that we cause to our bodies. Years of gorging on junk food, unhealthy lifestyle habits, and excessive sugar intake can not only make you gain weight but also lead to some serious health issues down the line. To relieve stress from our day-to-day lives, we often resort to eating habits that only give us temporary happiness. So what happens when your body can't take it any longer? You detox! Yes, a detox diet can be a lifesaver.

Though a human body is capable of detoxifying itself from time to time, drinking cleansing teas can certainly accelerate this process. Going on a detox tea cleanse diet drastically reduces your sugar cravings while keeping your energy high throughout the day. The extra hydration provided by detox teas can keep you feeling full for longer periods, thereby helping immensely in weight loss.

Let's look at how tea cleanse diet ingredients help your body.

GREEN TEA

Burns fat

Green tea is loaded with antioxidants, which assist in speeding up your body's metabolic rate. The faster your metabolism, the quicker you burn calories, thereby resulting in weight loss.

Improves immunity

Green tea can help you fight off all sort of common flu's colds and even sinus infections. It increases your body's disease-fighting capacity, thereby keeping most ailments at bay.

Re-hydration

If you are not used to at least 3-4 liters of water a day, green tea can keep you hydrated. Lack of hydration is known to lead to fatigue, lack of focus and a whole lot of other complications in your body. Drinking at least 2 cups of green tea a day will help you avoid any dehydration issues.

Wonder medicine

Research has proved that sipping on green tea daily can guard you against cancer, diabetes, neurological diseases like Alzheimer's and even arthritis.

HERBS & SPICES

Herbs can help in the elimination of the toxic built up in your body and reduce that heaviness in the belly. Wonder herbs & spices such as dandelion, ginger, pepper, fennel, cloves, cinnamon, cardamom and certain flowers can aid in offloading a lot of metabolic waste.

HONEY

Adding honey to your tea cleanse diets can provide you with plenty of vitamins and minerals. Raw honey is also packed with lots of antioxidants. Unlike refined sugar, honey does not add empty calories to your body, neither does it add to weight gain.

WHAT TO EXPECT POST A 7-DAYS TEA CLEANSE DIET?

How do you visualize yourself post the completion of your 7-day tea cleanse diet? A thinner version of yourself? Fully energized? Well, here are some more reasons.

- High energy levels
- No bloating
- No dehydration
- Weight loss
- Glowing skin
- Focused mind
- Increased stamina
- No stomach cramps
- Body will feel light

Chapter 2: detox routine, right type of teas and shopping list

Make detox teas a part of your lifestyle rather than indulging in them for a short period. Regularly sipping on such cleansing teas will help you maintain a stable weight throughout your life. One should also know what kind of tea you should indulge in at different times of the day. Here's what we recommend.

MORNING

During the morning, it's preferable to drink a cleansing tea that has ginger, lemon or turmeric added to it. Adding these ingredients will provide a great kick-start to your metabolism while keeping you refreshed for a longer duration. You can also indulge in smoothies during your breakfast, which will keep the hunger cravings at bay.

DAY

You can sip on multiple cups of plain green tea or teas that are blended with flower petals. You can also add your choice of herbs or spices to the drink to make it more energizing.

NIGHT

At night, you should focus on teas that can help you cleanse the colon. Teas like herbal tea or Ayurvedic tea can ensure flushing out of any toxic waste from your colon.

TEA CLEANSE SHOPPING LIST

If this is the first time you are planning to go on a tea cleanse diet, it is important for you to stock up the required ingredients from the supermarket. Try to buy fresh ingredients as much as possible and ensure that they are not sprayed with chemicals. You can also buy organic ingredients from trusted e-commerce websites such as eBay or Amazon. Here's a list of items you would need.

- Fruits of all kinds
- Green veggies
- Nuts and seeds

- All sorts of spices, herbs, and condiments
- Dairy products
- Almond milk
- Light coconut milk
- Rice milk
- Low-fat yogurt
- Chocolates & cocoa
- Dark cocoa powder (unsweetened and at least 85% cocoa)
- Sweeteners
- Raw Honey
- Maple syrup
- Agave
- Stevia
- Types of oils
- Olive oil
- Virgin coconut oil
- Flax seed oil
- Sesame oil
- Proteins
- Chicken

- Lamb
- Turkey
- Fish
- Sardines
- Salmon
- Black cod
- Trout
- Grains
- Whole wheat
- Quinoa
- Brown rice
- Wild rice

Chapter 3: tea cleanse diet meal plan

When you think about a 7-day diet schedule, you instantly imagine the uncontrollable hunger cravings one has to go through. The very thought of starving yourself for seven days in a row is incredibly overwhelming. The 7-day tea cleanse diet, on the other hand, can completely keep your hunger cravings at bay while keeping you energized throughout the week. This diet ensures that all the toxins are flushed out from your body while keeping you refreshed all the time.

Tea cleanse diet does not mean that one needs to drink only tea. It requires you to eat healthy and substantial meals while sipping on some yummy teas. The tea cleanse diet also consists of some smoothies to keep your tummy feeling full in the morning. This 7-day meal plan will give your belly the much-needed break from all the junk food you eat during the week. Also, we highly recommend you to stay away from caffeinated drinks as well as alcohol during this 7-day plan.

We have carefully chalked out a 7-day diet plan, which will help you shed off excess weight while detoxifying your body at the same time. If you happen to be a working professional, you can stock up all the ingredients a week ahead of your diet plan.

DAY 1

Pre-breakfast - Vitamin C herbal fusion tea

Breakfast - Egg and ham sandwich in brown bread

Lunch - Raw vegetables with smoked salmon and brown rice

Dinner - Vegetable stew along with smoked chicken breasts

DAY 2

Pre-breakfast - Rose petal and vanilla tea

Breakfast - Green tea almond and blueberry smoothie

Lunch - Quinoa with cooked vegetables and chicken salad

Dinner - Tuna with Chickpeas, Olives, and Romaine Lettuce Salad

DAY 3

Pre-Breakfast 2 - Soothing lemon tisane

Breakfast - Love your greens juice

Lunch - Tuna Lettuce Wraps with couscous

Dinner - Mexican Salad with Corn, Avocado, Beans, and Lime

DAY 4

Pre-Breakfast 2 - Apple green tea and turmeric tonic

Breakfast - Green Tea kiwi and mango smoothie

Lunch - Seared Shrimp in Coconut Oil with wild rice

Dinner - Spaghetti Squash with Garlic, Mushrooms & Tomato

DAY 5

Pre-Breakfast 2 - Refreshing Orange tea

Breakfast - Pumpkin-hazelnut Tea Soup

Lunch - Pineapple Chicken with stir-fried veggies

Dinner - Paleo Turkey Pesto Meatballs

DAY 6

Pre-Breakfast 2 - Acai & Strawberry Tea

Breakfast - Immune boosting strawberry smoothie

Lunch - Brown rice and mushroom risotto with cucumber salad

Dinner - Zucchini Stuffed Meatloaf

DAY 7

Pre-Breakfast 2 - Dandelion root detox tea

Breakfast - Detox Cactus Smoothie

Lunch - Brown rice and mushroom risotto with cucumber salad

Dinner - Aubergine Turkey Chili Sweet Potato

Chapter 4: tea cleanse recipes

LOVE YOUR GREENS JUICE

Serves: 2

Calories per serving: 145

Ingredients

- 4 cups baby spinach
- About 7-8 collard greens
- 1 large cucumber
- 1 small cup fresh parsley
- 1 small cup cilantro
- 2 tablespoon lemon juice
- Some ground pepper

Direction

1.   Wash the baby spinach and collard greens thoroughly under running water.

2.   Add them in a blender.

3.   Peel the cucumber skin off and slice it up roughly using a kitchen knife. Add it to the blender.

4. Slide in some parsley leaves and cilantro. Sprinkle some lemon juice and blend the mixture until smooth.

5. Pour into large glasses and serve with some ground pepper on top.

AYURVEDA DETOX TEA

Serves: 2

Calories per serving: 50

Ingredients

- ½ teaspoon cumin
- ½ teaspoon whole coriander
- 1 teaspoon whole fennel
- 5 cardamom pods
- 1 teaspoon honey
- 2 large glasses of water

Directions

1. Fill a vessel with some water and bring it to a boil.

2. Add all the above ingredients and stir using a spoon.

3. Let the mixture simmer for 15 minutes. Switch off the flame and cover the vessel with a lid. Let it stand for another 5 minutes.

4.   Sip on the tea on an empty stomach for better results

CLEANSING TEA

Serves: 4

Calories per serving: 63

Ingredients

- 1 half-inch cinnamon stick
- 2 tablespoons coriander seeds
- 1 small cup fresh cilantro
- ½ cup rosemary
- 2 inches peeled ginger
- 2 bags green tea
- 2 tablespoon honey
- 1 tablespoon apple cider vinegar
- About 5 cups of water

Directions

1.   Heat a saucepan over a slow flame and slightly toast the cinnamon stick until it starts releasing fragrance

2.   Fill a pot with some water and bring it to a boil.

3.   Slightly pound the ginger root and add it to the water.

4.   Add rest of the ingredients and let the mixture simmer for 15-20 minutes. Remove from flame and let the mixture stand for a few more minutes.

5.   Strain using a strainer and pour into large glasses.

6.   Serve hot.

ICED TURMERIC TEA

Serves: 2

Calories per serving: 24

Ingredients

- 2 cups water (around 500 ml)
- 1 1-inch ginger root, minced
- 2 teaspoons turmeric powder
- 2 green tea bags
- ¼ teaspoon salt
- 4 tablespoons honey
- Some ice cubes
- Fresh lime slices

Method

1. Fill a large pot with some water and bring it to a boil.

2. Add minced ginger, turmeric powder, honey, salt and mix well using a spoon.

3.   Let the mixture simmer for about 15 minutes on low heat.

4.   Dip the green tea bags in it and let the tea soak in.

5.   Strain using a strainer and fill into large teacups. Add 2 tablespoons honey to each cup and stir.

6.   Add ice cubes and garnish with some lemon slices on top and serve.

CHARCOAL TEA

Serves: 4

Calories per serving: 26

Ingredients

- 4 cups water
- 1 capsule of activated charcoal (about ¼ teaspoon)
- 3 tablespoons lemon juice
- 4 tablespoons honey
- ¼ teaspoon cardamom powder

Method

1. Fill a large vessel with about 4 cups of water and bring it to a boil.

2. Add lemon juice, cardamom powder, and activated charcoal powder and stir well using a wooden spoon.

3. Let the mixture simmer for 2-3 minutes. Remove from flame.

4. Add honey to the mixture and stir again.

5.   Strain using a strainer and serve in large cups.

LAVENDER AND LEMON TEA

Serves: 4

Calories per serving: 29

Ingredients

- 2 tablespoons lavender flowers
- Around 25 drops of stevia
- 4 cups water
- Some ice cubes
- 1 star anise
- Juice of half a lemon

Method

1. Fill a vessel with one cup of water and bring it boil.

2. Stir in the lavender flowers along with the star anise and let it seep in for about 15 minutes.

3. Add some lemon juice to a pitcher. Pour the remaining water along with some stevia and stir well.

4.   Pour the lavender mixture into the pitcher and mix all the ingredients using a spoon. Strain using a strainer and pour into large glasses.

5.   Serve along with some ice cubes.

IMMUNE BOOSTING STRAWBERRY SMOOTHIE

Serves: 2

Calories per serving: 65

Ingredients

- 1 large ripe banana
- 2 small cup fresh strawberries
- 1 small beet, peeled and diced
- 1 cup coconut water
- 2 tablespoons lime juice
- 4-5 ice cubes

Method

1.   Peel the banana and roughly chop it up using a kitchen knife.

2.   Add the banana slices to a blender along with some fresh strawberries and beet slices. Give it a whisk until you notice a smooth paste.

3.	Add coconut water, some lime juice and blend it again. Ensure there are no lumps.

4.	Pour into large glasses and add some ice cubes for a cooling effect.

5.	Serve chilled.

DETOX CACTUS SMOOTHIE

Serves: 5

Calories per serving: 60

Ingredients

- 2 medium sized cactus leaves
- 2 cups pineapple slices
- 2 medium bananas, peeled and sliced
- 1 cup Greek yogurt
- 4 tablespoons lime juice
- 2 cups almond milk
- 2 tablespoons honey (optional)

Method

1. Wash the cactus leaves thoroughly and carefully; remove the needles. Roughly chop them up using a sharp kitchen knife.

2. Add the cactus pieces to a blender followed by pineapple slices, banana slices, yogurt, honey, lime juice and whisk for a minute.

3.   Pour the almond milk into the blender and whisk again until it forms a smooth paste.

4.   Pour into large glasses and refrigerate for 2 hours before serving. You can also add some ice cubes instead.

RED CLOVER TEA

Serves: 4

Calories per serving: 32

Ingredients

- 1 cup red clover blossoms
- 2 teaspoons mint
- 4 cup of water
- 3 tablespoons honey
- 1 clove
- Some crushed ice

Method

1. Check for bugs while buying the red clover blossoms and make sure they aren't sprayed.
2. Fill some water in a large vessel. Add some red clover flowers to it and bring the water to a boil.
3. Add clove along with some mint and switch off the flame. Let it steep for 15 minutes and then strain through a strainer.

4. Add some honey and give the mixture a good stir.

5. Slide in some crushed ice and serve chilled.

CAYENNE PEPPER TEA

Serves: 2

Calories per serving: 33

Ingredients

- 2 green tea bags
- 2 ½ cups of water
- ½ teaspoon cayenne pepper
- ½ teaspoon turmeric
- 1 teaspoon lemon juice
- 1 1-inch cinnamon stick
- 1 tablespoon honey (optional)

Method

1. Boil around 2 cups of water in a large vessel. Now sprinkle some cayenne pepper, turmeric powder, lemon juice and stir.

2. Add cinnamon stick and simmer the mixture for about 10 minutes on low heat. Remove from flame once done.

3.   Dip the tea bags and let the mixture steep for 10 minutes.

4.   Strain using a strainer and add some honey. Stir well.

5.   Serve hot or add some crushed ice if you like it chilled.

AUTUMN TEA

Serves: 4

Calories per serving: 30

Ingredients

- 4 cups of water
- ½ cup red clover blossoms
- 1 1-inch ginger root
- 3-4 spearmint leaves
- ¼ teaspoon rosemary
- Thin slices of half a lemon

Method

1.   Fill a large vessel with about 4 cups of water and bring it to a boil.

2.   Throw in the red clover flowers along with some rosemary and simmer for 2-3 minutes on low flame.

3.   Gently pound the ginger and add it to the vessel. Throw in the spearmint leaves and simmer for another 3 minutes.

4.   Add the lemon slices to the mixture and let it steep for 10 minutes.

5.   Strain the mixture using a strainer and fill into large glasses.

6.   Serve hot.

HIBISCUS TEA

Serves: 4

Calories per serving: 38

Ingredients

- 5 teaspoons green tea bags
- 5 teaspoons chamomile
- ½ cup hibiscus flowers
- ½ cup orange peels or 2 tablespoons orange peel powder
- 8 teaspoons stevia
- 2 dried raspberries
- 4 tablespoons honey (optional)

Method

1. Add some water to a large vessel and bring it to a boil.

2. Throw in the hibiscus flowers, orange peels, raspberries, and stevia and let the mixture simmer for 10-12 minutes. Remove from flame once done.

3.   Dip the green tea bags in the mixture and let it steep for 8-10 minutes.

4.   Strain the tea through a strainer and add some honey to it. Stir well using a spoon.

5.   Pour into large cups and serve.

BLACK APPLE TEA

Serves: 2

Calories per serving: 51

Ingredients

- 1 large apple
- 2 tablespoons lemon juice
- 2 tablespoons honey
- 2-3 cloves
- 3 teaspoons leaf black tea
- 2 cinnamon sticks

Method

1. Wash the apples thoroughly under running water and pat them dry.

2. Peel the skin off using a peeler and cut the apple into thin slices.

3. Preheat the oven to 200 degrees C.

4.   Lay the apple slices on a greased tray and bake them for 20-25 minutes. Once cooled down, set them aside in a bowl.

5.   Boil some water in a large vessel and add the apple slices to it.

6.   Sprinkle some black tea into the water along with some cloves, cinnamon sticks and let the mixture simmer for 15 minutes.

7.   Remove from flame and strain with a strainer. Add honey and give it a stir.

8.   Serve hot.

SCHISANDRA FIVE FLAVOR TEA

Serves: 5 cups

Calories per serving: 58

Ingredients

- 2 tablespoons schisandra berries
- 4 small pieces of licorice root, pieced
- 3-inch ginger root, slightly pounded
- 2 tablespoons stevia
- 1 large cinnamon stick
- 5-6 eleuthero leaves
- 6 cups of water
- Some ice cubes

Method

1.   In a bowl, combine all the ingredients except for stevia and stir well using a large wooden spoon.

2.   Transfer this mixture to a large vessel and bring it to a boil.

3.   Lower the flame and add the stevia leaves.

4.   Cover with a lid and let the mixture simmer for 15-16 minutes.

5.   Strain the mixture using a large strainer and add it to a pitcher.

6.   Add some ice cubes and pour into large glasses.

7.   Serve chilled.

ELDERBERRY TEA

Serves: 2

Calories per serving: 44

Ingredients

- 2 large cups of water
- 1 1-inch cinnamon stick
- 2 small cardamom pods
- 2 cloves
- 2 large tablespoons of honey
- 2 tablespoons of dried elderberries

Method

1. Add some water to a saucepan and bring it to a boil.

2. Slightly pound the cardamom pods with a pounder and add them to the saucepan.

3. Add the elderberries, cloves, and cinnamon stick and stir well. Let the mixture simmer for 15 minutes.

4.   Strain the mixture through a strainer into teacups.

5.   Add about a tablespoon of honey to each of the two cups and stir.

6.   Serve hot.

HERBY TEA FOR A HAPPY TUMMY

Serves: 4

Calories per serving: 39

Ingredients

- 5 cardamom pods
- 1 teaspoon peppercorns
- 1 tablespoon fennel seeds
- 1 teaspoon coriander seeds
- 4-5 cloves
- 2 sticks of cinnamon
- 2 tablespoons minced ginger
- 4 teaspoons loose tea

Method

1.   Preheat the oven to 175 degrees C.

2.   Combine all the spices together in a bowl except tea and ginger.

3.   Lay the spices on a baking sheet and bake them for 5 minutes until they start releasing a fragrance.

4.   Add these toasted spices to some water along with some ginger and bring it to a boil.

5.   Add the tea powder and let the mixture simmer for 15 minutes.

6.   Pour in large cups and serve hot.

DANDELION ROOT DETOX TEA

Serves: 2

Calories per serving: 66

Ingredients

- 2 teaspoons dandelion root tea
- 2 tablespoons lemon juice
- 2 tablespoons fresh cranberry juice (without sugar)
- 1 tablespoons honey
- 2-3 cloves
- 2 cups water

Method

1. Fill a vessel with 2 cups of water and bring it to a boil.

2. Lower the flame and add dandelion tea powder and cloves to it. Simmer for 10 minutes.

3. Sprinkle some fresh lemon juice, followed by cranberry juice and honey. Stir the mixture using a spoon and simmer the mixture again for 5 minutes.

4. Strain the tea using a strainer and pour into large teacups.

5. Serve hot.

HERBY CHAI TEA

Calories per serving: 40

Serves: 4

Ingredients

- 4 cloves
- 4 cardamom pods
- 1 2-inch cinnamon stick
- 5-6 peppercorns
- 1 tablespoon fennels seeds
- 1 tablespoon dried ginger powder
- 2 star anise cloves
- 4 cups water
- 4 black tea bags

Method

1. Heat a saucepan and add all the above ingredients to it except water, tea bags and ginger powder.

2.   Toast all the spices on low heat for about 10-12 minutes until they start releasing flavor. Ensure that you keep stirring them occasionally. Once done, remove from flame.

3.   Add all the spices in a thick bowl and pound them with a pounder. You can also put them in a blender and make a smooth powder.

4.   Boil some water in a large vessel and add all the spice powder along with the dry ginger powder. Let the mixture simmer for 10-12 minutes on medium heat.

5.   Switch off the flame and dip the tea bags in the vessel. Let it steep for about 10 minutes.

6.   Strain the mixture using a strainer and pour into large cups.

7.   Serve hot.

GINGER TEA

Serves: 2

Calories per serving: 30

Ingredients

- 3 cups of water
- 1 1-inch ginger root
- 1 teaspoon ground turmeric
- Juice of one lemon
- 1 clove
- 2 tablespoons honey (optional)

Method

1. Fill a large vessel with about 2.5-3 cups of water and bring it to a boil.

2. Slightly pound the ginger root using a pounder and add it to the vessel.

3. Add turmeric powder, along and lemon juice to the vessel and stir using a spoon.

4.   Let the mixture simmer for 10-12 minutes on medium heat.

5.   Strain the mixture using a strainer and pour into teacups.

6.   Add a tablespoon of honey to each of these cups and stir.

7.   Serve hot.

CLEANSING TEA FOR WINTER

Serves: 4

Calories per serving: 52

Ingredients

- 4 cups water
- 1 2-inch cinnamon stick
- 1 tablespoon fennel seeds
- 1 tablespoon rose hips
- 6-7 cloves
- 2 small astralagus root pieces
- 6-7 peppercorns
- 3 tablespoons honey
- 1 cup skimmed milk (optional)

Method

1.   Fill a vessel with 4 cups of water and bring to a boil.

2.   Throw in the cinnamon sticks followed by fennel seeds, peppercorns, rose hips, and cloves and let it simmer for 10 minutes.

3.   Slightly pound the astralagus root pieces with a heavy object and add them to the vessel.

4.   Simmer the mixture for another 5-6 minute on low heat.

5.   Strain the mixture using a strainer.

6.   Pour some low-fat milk to the vessel along with some honey and stir using a spoon.

7.   Serve hot.

APPLE GREEN TEA AND TURMERIC TONIC

Calories per serving: 49

Serves: 4

Ingredients

- 4 ½ cups water
- 1 large green apple
- 2 1-inch cinnamon sticks
- 1 teaspoon organic turmeric powder
- 1 2-inch ginger root
- 2 teaspoons virgin coconut oil
- ¼ teaspoon cayenne pepper
- 3 green tea bags
- 2 tablespoons lemon juice
- 2 tablespoons honey

Method

1.   Wash the apple thoroughly under running water and pat it dry. Peel the skin off the slice it up using a knife.

2.   Fill a pan with some water and bring it to a boil.

3.   Throw in the apple slices into the vessel. Add turmeric powder, cayenne pepper, cinnamon sticks and stir well. Let it simmer for 10 minutes.

4.   Slightly pound the ginger root and add it to the vessel. Simmer gain for 5 more minutes. Switch off the flame.

5.   Dip the tea bags and let them steep for 10 minutes.

6.   Strain using a strainer into another vessel. Add coconut oil, honey and stir well.

7.   Pour the mixture into teacups and serve. You can reheat the tea if you like it hot.

ROSE PETAL AND VANILLA TEA

Serves: 4

Calories per serving: 26

Ingredients

- 4 tablespoons dried rose petals
- 1 large vanilla pod
- 4 cups water
- 2 tablespoons honey

Method

1.   Using a knife, carefully rip open the vanilla pod to take out the vanilla beans. Set aside.

2.   Boil some water in a large vessel.

3.   Lower the flame and add the vanilla beans along with dried rose petal and let the mixture simmer for 15 minutes on low flame.

4.   Strain the mixture using a strainer into a large pitcher. Add some honey and mix the tea well using a large spoon.

5.   Pour into large teacups and serve.

TRANQUIL TEA

Serves: 3

Calories per serving: 24

Ingredients

- 4 part chamomile
- 2 teaspoons dried lemon grass
- 2 teaspoons dried rose petals
- 1 teaspoon lemon juice
- 2 tablespoons honey

Method

1. Add all the herbs to a small glass bottle and shake them well until they are properly mixed.

2. Take some water in a large saucepan and bring it to a boil.

3. Lower the flame and add all the spices from the bottle.

4. Let the tea simmer for 12-15 minutes on low heat.

5.   Strain the mixture carefully into a pitcher.

6.   Add about 2 tablespoons honey to the pitcher and mix well.

7.   Pour into teacups and serve.

FEMININE BALANCE TEA

Serves: 4

Calories per serving: 47

Ingredients

- 4 ½ cups of tea
- 1 tablespoon red clover blossoms
- 1 tablespoon dried raspberry leaves
- 2 tablespoons fennel seeds
- 1 teaspoon dried orange peel powder
- 3-4 hibiscus flower petals
- ½ teaspoon vitex
- 3 tablespoons raw honey
- Some crushed ice

Method

1. Boil about 4 ½ cups of water in a large saucepan.

2. Add red clover blossoms, dried raspberry leaves, fennel seeds, orange peel powder, hibiscus flower petals and stir well using a large wooden spoon.

3.   Let the mixture simmer for 8-9 minutes.

4.   Add vitex and simmer for 2-3 minutes more.

5.   Strain the tea into a large pitcher using a strainer.

6.   Add 3 tablespoons honey and stir again. Remove from flame and let it cool down.

7.   Add some crushed ice to the tea and pour into large cups.

8.   Serve chilled.

SERENDIPI TEA

Serves: 4

Calories per serving: 52

Ingredients

- 7-8 spearmint leaves
- 1 teaspoon peppermint
- 2 tablespoons chamomile blossoms
- ¾ teaspoon lemon balm
- 1 teaspoon dried rose petals
- Leaves of one blue cornflower
- 2 tablespoons honey
- 4 cups water

Method

1.   Combine all the herbs in a small bowl and mix well.

2.   Boil about 4 cups of water in a large vessel. Once it comes to a boil, lower the flame.

3.   Add the mixed herbs and simmer the tea for 15 minutes on low heat or 8 minutes on high.

4.   Add two tablespoons honey to the vessel and switch off the flame. Let the tea steep for 6-7 minutes.

5.   Strain into a large pitcher using a strainer.

6.   Pour into large teacups and serve.

REFRESHING KOMBUCHA TEA

Serves: 4

Calories per serving: 40

Ingredients

- 3 cups of distilled water
- 2 green tea bags
- 2 black tea bags
- 5-6 mint leaves
- 2 teaspoons brown sugar (you can use honey too, but it makes the tea slightly sticky)
- ¾ cup Kombucha (store-bought)
- 1 large SCOBY

Method

1. Fill a vessel with about 4 cups of water and bring it to a boil.

2. Add mint leaves, brown sugar and tea bags.

3. Allow the mixture to steep for about 20 minutes.

4. Stir the mixture properly so that the brown sugar gets dissolved completely.

5. Pour the mixture into a large pitcher.

6. Once it cools down, add the Kombucha and SCOBY.

7. Now cover the pitcher with a muslin cloth and secure it with a rubber band.

8. Place the pitcher in a room with a consistent temperature for about 5 days.

9. Once it's fermented, you can strain, add some ice cubes and pour into large cups.

10. Serve chilled.

PUMPKIN-HAZELNUT TEA SOUP

Serves: 4

Calories per serving: 42

Ingredients

- 4 cups of water
- 3 hazelnut tea sachets
- 3 small cups of roasted pumpkin puree
- 3 tablespoons honey
- ¼ teaspoon salt
- 2 tablespoons dry hazelnuts
- 1 teaspoon minced ginger

Method

1. Boil some water in a large vessel.

2. Lower the flame and add hazelnut tea sachets. Simmer the tea for 12-14 minutes on medium flame.

3. Pour the pumpkin puree into the vessel followed by some salt, minced ginger and stir well using a spoon. Let it steep for 7-8 minutes.

4.   In the meanwhile, roughly chop the hazelnuts and slightly toast them on a saucepan. Set aside.

5.   Strain the tea using a strainer into a pitcher.

6.   Add honey and stir.

7.   Pour into teacups and garnish with toasted hazelnuts.

ACAI & STRAWBERRY TEA

Serves: 8 cups

Calories per serving: 24

Ingredients

- 8 cups water
- ½ cup fresh mint
- 2 small cups of frozen strawberries
- 6 bags of acai berry tea
- 4 green tea bags
- 5 tablespoons honey

Method

1. Fill a saucepan with some distilled water and bring it to a boil over high flame.

2. Lower the flame and dip the tea bags. Boil for another 5-6 minute on medium flame.

3. Transfer the tea to a large pitcher.

4. Roughly chop up some strawberries and add to the pitcher.

5. Add mint leaves, honey, and mix well.

6. Let it steep for 15 minutes and strain using a strainer.

7. Add crushed ice and pour into large teacups and serve.

REFRESHING ORANGE TEA

Serves: 4

Calories per serving: 34

Ingredients

- 1 large cup fresh orange juice (without sugar)
- 4 tablespoons honey
- ¼ teaspoon cayenne pepper
- 2-3 cloves
- 4 slices of lemon for garnishing
- 4 cups of water
- 4 tea bags
- Basil sprigs
- Some ice cubes

Method

1.   Fill a saucepan with some water and bring it to a boil.

2.   Add orange juice, honey, pepper, cloves and boil for another 5 minutes on low heat.

3.	Dip the tea bags and simmer the mixture for 5 minutes.

4.	Switch off the flame and let the tea steep for 10 minutes. Add honey and stir well.

5.	Strain through a strainer into large cups.

6.	Add some ice cubes and garnish them with lemon slices on the edge of the glasses.

7.	Slightly rub the basil leaves in between your palms, so it releases flavor.

8.	Sprinkle them on top and serve.

VITAMIN C HERBAL FUSION TEA

Serves: 4

Calories per serving: 30

Ingredients

- 4 tablespoons rose hips
- 1 tablespoon lemongrass
- 1 tablespoon broken cinnamon chips
- 4-5 hibiscus flower petals
- 1 tablespoon fennel seeds
- 4 cups water
- Some ice cubes
- 2 tablespoons honey (optional)

Method

1. Combine all the herbs in a small jar. Close the lid and shake them well, so they get mixed properly.

2. Boil about 4 cups of water in a large saucepan.

3. Add the above herbs and boil again for about 5-7 minutes.

4. Remove from flame and cover with a lid. Let the mixture steep for at least 30 minutes, so the flavors are completely released.

5. Add honey and stir with a spoon.

6. You can refrigerate the tea for a couple of hours or add crushed ice and serve.

SOOTHING LEMON TISANE

Serves: 4 cups

Calories per serving: 25

Ingredients

- 3 teaspoons lemon grass
- 1 teaspoon lemon balm
- Peels of one lemon
- 1 teaspoon chamomile
- ¼ teaspoon stevia
- 2 cloves
- 4 cups water

Method

1. Fill a large pot with some distilled water and bring it to a boil.

2. To this, add lemon grass, lemon balm, lemon peels, chamomile, cloves and boil for 10 more minutes on low heat.

3.   Add stevia and stir the mixture with the help of a spoon.

4.   Cover the lid and let the mixture steep for 15 minutes.

5.   Add stevia and mix well.

6.   Remove from flame and strain using a strainer.

7.   Serve hot.

GREEN TEA KIWI AND MANGO SMOOTHIE

Serves: 4

Calories per serving: 65

Ingredients

- 2 ripe mangoes, diced
- ¾ cup fat-free yogurt
- ¼ cup honey
- 2 small ripe kiwis, peeled and sliced
- 2 tablespoons green tea
- 1 cup water
- Some ice cubes

Method

1. Boil some water in a large vessel.

2. Add green tea powder and boil for another 7-8 minute. Switch off the flame and let it steep for 10 minutes.

3. Strain using a strainer into a pitcher. Set aside.

4.   In a blender, add the mango slices followed by kiwi, honey and give it a whisk.

5.   Add the yogurt and whisk again until forms a smooth paste.

6.   Pour the green tea in the blender along with some honey.

7.   Pour into large cups and add some crushed ice on top.

8.   Serve chilled.

GREEN TEA ALMOND AND BLUEBERRY SMOOTHIE

Serves: 3

Calories per serving: 55

Ingredients

- 2 green tea bags
- 1 cup fat-free yogurt
- 2 small cups blueberries
- 2 tablespoons flaxseeds
- 1 tablespoon virgin coconut oil
- 3 cups water
- Some ice cubes
- Some mint sprigs
- 3-4 strawberries thinly sliced for garnishing
- 5-6 roasted almonds

Method

1. Boil some water in a large vessel.

2.   Add green tea powder and boil for another 7-8 minute. Switch off the flame and let it steep for 10 minutes.

3.   Strain using a strainer into a pitcher. Set aside.

4.   In a blender, add blueberries, flax seeds, yogurt, and coconut oil and give it a whisk. Ensure there are no lumps in the mixture.

5.   Transfer into a large pitcher. Now pour the green tea into it and mix well using a spoon.

6.   Pour the tea into large glasses.

7.   Add some ice cubes on top

8.   Garnish with sliced strawberries carefully tucked onto the edge of the glasses.

9.   Roughly chop up the almonds, add them on top and serve.

MINTY PEACH TEA

Serves: 4

Calories per serving: 25

Ingredients

- About 10 mint leaves
- 2 ripe peaches
- 2 cloves
- 2 tablespoons honey
- ½ teaspoon minced ginger
- 4 cups of water
- Some crushed ice

Method

1. Wash the peaches thoroughly and pat them dry. Peel the skin off and dice them.

2. Fill a large saucepan with about 4 cups of water and bring it to a boil.

3. Slide in the sliced peaches along with some cloves, minced ginger, mint, leaves and boil for another 7-8 minute on low heat.

4. Cover the lid and let the mixture steep for 20 minutes.

5. Strain using a strainer into a jar. Add honey and stir well with a spoon.

6. Refrigerate for 2 hours or add some crushed ice cubes and serve.

Conclusion

Thank you once again for choosing this book. Aren't the recipes in the book much simpler and more fun than you thought? We knew you would enjoy reading them as much as we enjoyed writing them for you. By following this diet, you would not only end up knocking off a few pounds but you will also notice how hydrated your skin becomes. Flushing out the toxins can help the body cleanse itself and bounce back with renewed energy.

Part 2

Introduction

This book has actionable steps and strategies on how to find and choose the best teas to cleanse your body, the benefits of tea as part of a lifestyle, and a 1-week plan for overall health and well being.

So why should you go on a tea cleanse? Well, simple; tea detox is a gentle way to detox your body since it involves adding a few cups of herbal tea to your diet, unlike other detox formulas that ask for the replacement of your meals entirely. Furthermore, basic herbal and black teas are rich in antioxidants, which is the secret behind boosting the natural cleansing process.

So, why detox, when the body can naturally cleanse itself?

Tea detoxification can help you remove toxins naturally from your body while helping you maintain healthy weight. These toxins may include pollutants, pesticides, and chemicals. Our bodies are designed to rid themselves of these toxins naturally but most of the time our detox process is overburdened so the body cannot detox itself fully. Because of this, it is critical to cleanse because these toxins can contribute to:

- Food cravings and weight gain

- Problems with your digestive tract

- Fatigue and difficulty sleeping

- Congestion

- Reduced mental clarity

- Low libido

- Skin issues

- Joint discomfort

As such, it is very important that we do something about our high levels of toxicity if we are to live a healthy life free from the complications we've mentioned above. Nature has given us wonderful tools to use. One way to make this possible is to detox using tea. If you are wondering how this works and how to go about it, this book will teach you all that in an easy to follow structure. But as a rule of thumb, it is important to consult your doctor or healthcare provider before starting any new diet plan, especially if you have caffeine sensitivities, as many varieties are caffeinated. If this is you, you can still benefit from the numerous un-caffeinated herbal tea recipes inside.

Thank you again for downloading this book, I hope you enjoy it!

Chapter 1: tea basics
HOW TEA IS GROWN

Though tea can be grown in many environments, the best place to grow traditional tea plants is in cooler climates with high altitudes. Tea plants fare best in acidic soil and regions with heavy rainfall.

In the early stages, the tea plant is pruned constantly. When the tea plant reaches maturity, leaves can be harvested from it four to five times a year for many years. Harvest depends on when the plant begins to flush. The picking must begin at exactly the right time so that the leaves are large enough but not too old to ensure flavor and nutritional benefits. Most tea is picked by hand for better quality. This is because machines tend to be rough and end up damaging too many leaves.

Only the top two leaves and a bud are picked for the best green and black tea. Sometimes the bud alone is picked for specialty teas.

Once enough leaves are collected, they are quickly carried over to a tea factory. The tea is then processed for two main reasons: for the sake of preservation by driving out most of the moisture and to bring the flavor to the surface so that it can quickly transfer to the water during the steeping process. Depending on the type of tea product being made, the tea leaves may go through a variety of processes from simple drying to fermenting.

Organic vs. Non-organic tea

The organic label refers to the way teas are produced and grown. Organic teas are safe for your health and the environment. Teas grown organically, focus on conserving our environment and health by being cultivated free from synthetic fertilizers, herbicides and pesticides. Organic farming conserves water and soil. Organic tea is also not biogenetically engineered or genetically altered in any way.

Environmental damage caused by non-organic tea production

Non-organic farming of tea uses over a million pounds of pesticides every year. At least 13 pesticides are commonly used in tea production in India alone resulting in poisoning of the soil. Tea plants in commercial gardens require periodic fertilization because of the nutrients lost during the harvesting of the leaves. Heavy application of nitrogen in the tea fields causes soil acidification and serious contamination of local water with nitrates. As a result, the farmers have to use more chemicals to enrich the soil. This leads to increased environmental damage. If the residue from this system is left in processed tea, it can easily leach into your cup during brewing. The rate of leaching will vary from one pesticide to another. When they enter our system, they can potentially cause great damage. This is opposite of the goal we want to achieve in a tea cleanse, better health. It is this reason that we believe organic tea is better for your health than non-organic tea.

THE ART OF STEEPING

Steeping can make or break a cup of tea. The process begins when you pour heated water over the tea bag, tea strainer, or infuser, the goal of steeping being to infuse the water and the tea. You will extract the most pleasure from fine tea if you steep it with care. It is important to understand that different teas take different durations to steep and understanding this will make the difference between drinking a bland cup of tea and enjoying a great cup of tea. In addition, over steeping will cause bitterness. Therefore, it is important to experiment with different types of teas, (bags or lose leaf teas,) to know the appropriate steeping times of each. You will find a steep time guide in the information below.

The difference between steeping and brewing
Brewing and steeping are both a part-and-parcel of the same process. Brewing is the act of making tea and steeping is the process involved. Brewing a superb cup of tea relies on three main components: high-quality water, quality tea leaves and correct steeping time. The

rule of thumb for brewing a cup of tea consists of 1 teaspoon loose leaf tea or one tea bag. The exceptions are mild herbal, yellow, white, and Oolong teas that require 2 teaspoons of tea for better flavor and health benefit. Always use fresh spring or filtered water when brewing tea. You can optionally warm the cup before brewing by adding a little freshly boiled water, swirling, and pouring out.

Steeping to perfection

Green and white teas are more delicate and therefore, you should steep with water that is heated to just below the boiling point and for less time. You can steep heartier teas such as Oolong, red, black, and herbal varieties with water that has fully boiled without the worry of over processing. See the next page for a convenient, quick reference chart.

Tea Variety	Bagged Steep Time	Loose-Leaf Steep Time
White Tea	Around 1 minute	Up to 3 minutes

Green Tea	Around 3 minutes	Up to 4 minutes
Black Tea	Up to 5 minutes	Up to 5 minutes
Oolong Tea	Up to 7 minutes	Up to 7 minutes
Red and Herbal Teas	Up to 7 minutes	Up to 7 minutes

Loose-leaf tea is typically superior to tea bags in quality, freshness, taste and aroma. Loose-leaf tea offers economical value as well, extending further for more cups per package as compared to the tea bag, especially when brewing larger batches. Either is fine for the recipes you will find inside this book.

If using loose-leaf tea, you will need an infuser or a strainer to help remove the leaves from the tea once it reaches the desired steep time. When making a larger batch, a tea kettle is useful. Many have built in strainers. Delicate teas like green and white teas do well in a porcelain or glass kettle that is more likely to release heat. Black tea, Oolong, and herbal teas can handle the higher heat of an iron kettle. A french press is also very useful when making teas infused with other ingredients, such as the Ayurvedic teas found further in this chapter.

Steeped tea leaves have a lot of uses beyond the cup. Some options are as a deodorizer (a dried tea bag can help remove odors from shoes or the refridgerator), a nitrogen-rich addition to your compost pile, an exfoliant in homemade soaps, or even a smoking agent for meat or fish!

Chinese tea

Chinese people have enjoyed tea for millennia and it is therefore, greatly intertwined with Chinese culture. While many simply enjoyed its flavor, the nobility considered tea consumption to be a mark of status while scholars hailed the brew as a cure for a variety of ailments.

Ancient Chinese legend attributes Shen Nong, an early Chinese emperor and herbalist, as first discovering tea. According to folklore, one day while resting with his army, the emperor requested some freshly boiled water. Somewhere along the way, a dried leaf fell into the water altering its color. Not seeing the change in his water, the emperor drank his brew. Having enjoyed his drink, tea came into existence!

Camellia sinensis is the tea plant responsible for teas we are familiar with from both China and India. The camellia sinensis sinensis plant yields green, black, oolong, white, and yellow teas commonly consumed in China. This evergreen plant has glossy green leaves and small white flowers with cheery yellow centers. Most often, the plant is not allowed to flower so the bush will continue to produce buds and tender foliage for harvesting. When allowed to flower, the resulting fruit is a protective green shell around a single brown seed. The seeds can then be harvested to make tea seed oil, (not to be confused with tea tree oil from the melaleuca plant,) which is used for a variety of topical and internal benefits.

Green tea

Green tea is the oldest and most popular type of tea. It has been enjoyed in China for thousands of years. Made from the new shoots of tea plants, the leaves are dried and processed according to desired flavor and intensity. The traditional green tea has a pale color and a strong astringent flavor. This tea is known for its many health benefits including anti-inflammatory and detoxification properties, improved digestion and increased mental alertness.

Here is a sample green tea recipe that is delicious and satisfying in all seasons. The fruit additions below will help the new green tea drinker grow accustomed to its flavor as well as improve digestion and assist detoxification.

This and many other recipes can be made in large batches for easy consumption throughout the day. Please store in the refrigerator for maximum refreshment.

BREWING DETOX GREEN TEA

Ingredients

2 slices cucumber

2 strawberries sliced

1 teaspoon honey

1 slice lemon

1 green tea bag

Instructions

1.   Use the green tea bag and almost boiled water to brew 8-10 fluid ounces of green tea. Once the tea has steeped (3 minutes bagged or 4 minutes loose leaf), stir in the honey to dissolve.

2.   Chill the green tea for 5 minutes in the refrigerator, remove, and add lemon, cucumber, and strawberries. Add ice if desired then stir to mix.

Black tea

Black tea is made from new shoots of tea leaves that are wilted, rolled, fermented and dried. This infusion yields a lovely red color and a subtle aromatic fragrance. Black tea contains antioxidants, which look for cell damaging free radicals in the body and destroys them.

BREWING BLACK TEA

Ingredients

2 teaspoons loose leaf black tea

6 ounces water

Optional: fruit preserves, honey, lemon, and/or milk of choice

Instructions

1.   Heat water in a teakettle to a rolling boil.

2.   Place the tea leaves directly into the cup and pour the warm water in the same cup.

3.   Cover the cup with a small saucer.

4.   Set the timer for 3-5 minutes or until the tea is to your liking.

5.   Stop the infusion as soon as the tea is ready. Strain it into a cup to remove the leaves.

6.   Add milk, lemon or honey. Don't use lemon if you are using milk.

Oolong tea

Oolong tea is produced by exposing the leaves to the sun which causes oxidation and wilting. This results in a curly, twisted appearance. Oolong tea aids in fat decomposition by boosting your metabolism. As a beauty enhancer, the rich levels of antioxidants can prevent hair loss and add shine when used as a rinse. It's also know to stabilize blood glucose for those suffering with type 2 diabetes.

BREWING OOLONG TEA

Ingredients

2 tablespoons Oolong tea

6 ounces water

Instructions

1.   Heat water in a teakettle until boiling.

2.   Place the Oolong tea leaves in the cup. Pour the water over the tealeaves. Cover the cup with a small saucer. Allow the tea to steep for between 1-5 minutes. Taste the tea at 1 minute and then after every 30 seconds until it is to your liking.

3.   Stop the infusion as soon as the tea is ready and remove the leaves by pouring the tea through a strainer.

White tea

White tea is uncured, unfermented green tea that has been quickly dried. It has a subtle delicate flavor and has a lighter color than any other type of tea. Its rumored that it got its name from the tradition of poor Chinese, who if they had no tea, would offer plain boiled water to guests and call it 'white tea'. More likely, its name is due to the light color of the leaves once dried. The drink itself has a light yellow appearance. It has anti-aging properties, which help in maintaining good internal health. Topically, it has also been proven to protect the skin from the harmful effects of UV light.

BREWING WHITE TEA

Ingredients

2 teaspoons white tea per cup

6 ounces of water

Instructions

1.   Bring water to a rolling boil then remove from heat.

2.   Add 2 teaspoons of white tea in the warm cup and fill the cup with very hot spring water.

3.   Cover and steep for about 5 minutes.

4.   Strain the leaves from the tea and enjoy your cup of tea.

Yellow tea

Yellow Tea is produced by allowing tea leaves that are damp to naturally dry. It has a distinct aroma closer to that of black tea but with a flavor closer to white and green tea. Yellow tea aids in weight loss. Known to prevent certain types of cancer lately as a rich source of amino acids and polyphenols, it is also heart healthy in lowering blood pressure and cholesterol. The tea is in high demand because it is an excellent source of antioxidants and fluoride, which help to make bones stronger and prevent tooth decay.

BREWING YELLOW TEA

Ingredients

1 heaping teaspoon yellow tea per 250ml water

Porcelain teapot (preferred)

Instructions

1. Bring water to a rolling boil then remove from heat.

2. Place the tea leaves in the warm water pot. Steep for 60 seconds if it is the first infusion. You can make up to 3 infusions.

3. Arrange the cups in a circle and pour the brew out in a continuous circular motion. This will ensure the taste of the tea is perfectly balanced.

AYURVEDIC TEA

Ayurveda is an ancient Indian healing system which directly translated means "the science of life". It is of the belief that we are one unit and illness stems from an imbalance of the three energies of body, mind, and spirit. In Ayurvedic medicine, prevention is the leading guide that creates food and lifestyle routines specific to the individual's needs.

Ayurvedic medicine stems from ancient roots of India and has been in practice for over 5000 years. It emphasizes cleansing your body of impurities in order to promote good health. Ayurvedic teas are powerful teas, effective in balancing the digestive system by balancing the body's PH. These teas are herbal mixtures that include plants and spices effective in promoting health and longevity.

Camellia sinensis assamica is the native tea plant found in the Assam region of Northern India. It is a prolific grower and can be harvested every 8 to 12 days for making strong black teas. Left on its own, it can grow upwards of 60 feet with leaves reaching 8 inches in length.

Ayurvedic teas are a little extra-ordinary with kicks of spicy freshness and sweet fruitiness. Their combination of the most luxurious herbs is thought to help you stay younger for longer. This combination also regulates metabolism of fat, maintaining the level of fat in the body, correcting the metabolic rate and maintaining it. It removes excess fat from the blood to stop unnecessary fat entering and being stored in the body. Ayurvedic medicine is also beneficial in improving digestion and the overall functioning of your body. An inefficient digestive system is unable to remove all the harmful toxins from your body. The buildup of toxins can lead to indigestion and other diseases of the stomach. By improving on digestion, your body is able to remove all the excess toxins in your gastro-intestinal system. Improved digestion can also lead to faster weight loss and strengthened immunity.

Purchasing the spices used in the following recipes can be quite an investment. Rest assured that these not only will last you a long time, but their health benefits can be used in a variety of cooking recipes as well. When possible, purchase organic. Always store spices away from heat and moisture.

AYURVEDIC TEA, A DETOXING CHAI TEA

Ingredients

A squeeze of lemon

2 tablespoons green, black, or ginger tea

2 tablespoons fennel seeds

2 tablespoons cumin seeds

2 tablespoons coriander seeds

1 tablespoon thinly sliced fresh turmeric

2 tablespoons thinly sliced ginger

1 quart boiling water

Instructions

1.	Place all the ingredients in a French press and let it stand for 5 minutes before plunging and serving.

2.	Press can be refilled a second time using the ingredients for another infusion.

3.	Alternatively, simmer all the ingredients together for 5 minutes in a pot and strain before drinking.

BONUS RECIPE

GOLDEN MILK (TUMERIC MILK)

Tumeric is prized for its liver enzyme activating properties. Tumeric is also getting a lot of attention as a natural anti-inflammatory. Beneficial for both digestion and immune function, this simple milk is a delicious and powerful Ayurvedic addition to any of the hot teas brewed from this section.

Ingredients

1 cup milk of choice (animal or nut/seed milk)

½ teaspoon tumeric

¼ teaspoon cinnamon

1 teaspoon honey or maple syrup to taste

¼ teaspoon ginger (or an optional thumb of fresh ginger peeled and coined)

pinch of black pepper (to increase absorption)

optional pinch of cayenne pepper (if you do not mind the heat)

Heat all of the ingredients in a sauce pan until just boiling. Simmer for 5-10 minutes. Strain and serve immediately on it's own or as an added milk to your tea of choice.

Chapter 2: teas for stronger immunity

You may have heard it was an apple, but actually, a cup of tea a day can keep the doctor away. When you have a strong, well functioning immune system, it means not only that you will become sick less often, but also that whenever you become ill, you will benefit from a quicker recovery. In other words, your immune system is the gatekeeper to good health. It is your body's unique design to resist millions of viruses, toxins, microbes, bacteria and germs that we expose ourselves to every day. Because we cannot prevent our bodies from exposure to the millions of germs and viruses in our environment, it is important that we build our immune systems to protect us from any possible damage caused by disease. Eating healthy foods and drinking the right beverages for the sake of our immunity, is a wise daily investment we can make for our well being.

Green tea fights bacteria

Studies have revealed that taking about 3 cups of green tea a day can directly help prevent infection by fighting bacteria. This tea introduces 5 times the amount of anti-bacterial protein in your blood. The tea plant, camellia sinensis, naturally contains the amino acid L-theanine. L-theanine has shown a consistency in strengthening immunity, fighting off infection and most importantly increasing the level of gamma delta T cells. Gamma delta T is our body's first defense against infection. A simple way to get L-theanine is by including tea in our diet. Green tea, specifically matcha, has shown the exceptional ability to fight germs. L-theanine is also available in black, white and oolongs teas but in much smaller content.

The magic of matcha

Matcha is made from a high quality, Japanese green tea. Matcha is high in chlorophyll because during the period of growth, its leaves are shaded. Chlorophyll has an abundance of benefits such as aiding in blood clotting and wound healing. The shading also increases the level of L-theanine found in higher concentrations in young greens. At harvest, the leaves are plucked and laid out flat to dry. The veins are then removed and the leaves are ground until they become very fine ground powder with a consistency of talc. This keeps the powerful chlorophyll and L-theanine preserved.

Apart from building your immune system, matcha has natural fiber that helps to detoxify the body of toxins, improve digestion and help the body do its work of fighting off bacteria and viruses.

MATCHA TEA

Ingredients

1 teaspoon match for every 6 ounce cup of water

Heat water to just boiling and let rest a minute before steeping. Measure the powder and wisk while dry to remove clumps. Pour water over the tea and wisk one more time to fully incorporate. Powder stays in the cup, no straining necessary.

Optional add-ins: mint, lemon, honey, frothy milk for a latte, vanilla extract

Matcha powder is also great in a variety of recipes from ice creams to baked goods (and did I mention its a fun way to benefit from its powerful nature?).

Chapter 3: teas for inflammation

Inflammation is part of the body's natural immune defense. Unfortunately in our over stressed, over stimulated society, and poorly nourished society, its presence does more harm than good to our bodies. A good number of disorders and diseases are traced to chronic and severe inflammation. What's more, the foods that we eat may knowingly and unknowingly contain pro-inflammatory compounds that make the situation worse. As taxed as our systems are, teas can help assist in the detoxification and ultimately, inflammation-reducing process.

Teas naturally contain antioxidants. Younger leaves contain an even greater anti-oxidant content. Antioxidants essentially stop inflammation before it starts by preventing oxidative damage to our cells. Normally our body handles this process well but environmental and dietary factors can increase the need for assistance. Whole foods and teas are wonderful at helping this process.

Drinking tea can be a great complimentary treatment for arthritis, one of the diseases caused by inflammation. It will help lessen pain, ease joint stiffness, and even prevent the condition from getting worse. Some of the teas for inflammation include:

Ginger tea- this is a versatile aromatic spice with very strong anti-oxidant, anti-inflammatory, and analgesic properties. Ginger is easily available in the grocery store. Slice ginger and steep it in hot water or add it to your green tea.

Tumeric tea- tumeric's active ingredient, curcumin, is a powerful, natural anti-inflammatory. Use either recipe from the Ayurvedic section above for a delicious and effective inflammation reducing tea.

Green tea- a simple cup of green tea is full of quercetin, a bioflavanoid that is full of anti-inflammatory effects. Quercetin relieves rheumatoid arthritis and prevents damage of your joints.

Nettle leaf tea- the nettle leaf is covered with tiny stiff hairs, especially on its underside such that they produce a stinging chemical when touched. These chemicals have been proven to relieve pain by reducing the levels of anti-inflammatory chemicals. Steep one tablespoon dried stinging nettle with one cup of boiling water. Add sweetener, lemon, or mint if desired.

Chapter 4: teas for better digestion

Both green tea and herbal tea may help improve your digestion and limit any adverse digestive effects like stomach upset and gas. Because all teas are high in anti-inflammatory properties to some extent, the tea is likely to reduce your digestion problems if it caused by inflammation. Studies have revealed that black tea prevents pancreatitis by calming the production of amylase and lipase. These two enzymes are important in digestion and their regulation may reduce symptoms of certain types of conditions.

Green tea contains polyphenols including catechins. Catechins increase the activity of pepsin, the digestive enzyme that breaks down protein in the stomach. Green tea also protects the lining of your small intestines as it moves through your digestive system by refortifying depleted anti-oxidant levels to actually protect your body against the free radicals that come with stress. Both physical and emotional stress can be damaging to your digestion. Diseases like inflammatory bowel syndrome produce extra intestinal stress. Regular consumption of tea high in anti-oxidants can help mitigate the damage.

Chai tea contains a mixture of spices including ginger, cardamom, pepper, and cinnamon. Cinnamon helps relieve a variety of digestive ailments such as heartburn, indigestion, gas, nausea, and stomach crumps. Ginger may also improve digestion and relieve an upset stomach and nausea.

Dandelion tea has good laxative effects that make it excellent for constipation problems. It helps to make the bowel regular and laxative. A teaspoon of dried dandelion roots steeped in boiled water is good enough to improve digestion.

Peppermint tea is also known for soothing nausea and stomach upset. As a prolific grower, fresh peppermint is an inexpensive, readily available remedy for digestion issues. 7-10 fresh leaves steeped for 5 minutes in a cup of boiled water makes an aromatic and effective drink. Likewise, dried peppermint at one heaping teaspoon per cup of water will work well when fresh is not available.

Chapter 5: teas for brain health

Chemicals found in green tea, may prevent brain damage that occurs after strokes and other brain injuries. Caffeine is one of the basic components of green tea and has shown to improve brain functions through improvements in mood, memory, and reaction time. Another good thing about green tea is that it does not contain too much caffeine, like coffee, therefore helping you avoid that jittery and edgy feeling while benefitting from the other numerous benefits of its leaves.

Caffeine also blocks the neurotransmitter adenosine meaning that, the neurons fire more dopamine, and therefore norepinephrine is increased. The l-thianine amino acid present works in a process that has anti-anxiety effects. L-thianine helps in improving your mental health by working in conjunction with caffeine.

Lack of mental clarity can be caused by lack of sleep, substance abuse, stress, injury, depression and many others. For occasional mental fog, consider a hot cup of tea. This includes both real tea and herbal teas. Try one teaspoon of each of these in a cup of boiling water for improved mental function:

Ginko Biloba, which makes an excellent tea for memory retention and positive neurological effects.

Gotu Kola, which is popular for memory retention. Gotu kola works by improving blood circulation in our brains and in turn assisting you with better clarity, focus, concentration and an increased attention span.

Rhodiola rosea is a golden root herb whose tea, apart from improving focus and concentration, is associated with combating the symptoms of depression.

Chapter 6: teas for weight loss

Green tea has gained popularity for its ability to boost metabolism and aid in weight loss. Green tea is loaded with potent antioxidants referred to as catechins and the most important of them being EGCG, a substance, which usually boosts metabolism. Better metabolism means that you can burn 3-4% more calories each day.

Green tea also helps metabolize fats from fat cells. EGCG can help inhibit the enzyme that breaks down the hormone norepinephrine. When this enzyme is inhibited, the amount of norepinephrine is increased. This hormones act as a signal to your hormones telling them to break down fat cells. This increases the release of fats into the bloodstream and makes it readily available as energy by the muscles that need it. Weight loss comes about when this fat is burnt for energy instead of being stored. Apart from green tea, other teas for weight loss are:

White tea- this is because it prevents the formation of new fat cells while helping to break down some.

Remember, it is the least processed tea making it a rich source of anti-oxidants, even more than green tea.

Rooibos tea- this comes from the leaves of the 'red bush' plant found in South Africa. What makes it good for your belly is Aspalathin, a unique and powerful flavonoid that can reduce stress hormones, which usually trigger hunger along with storage of fats. Rooibos is a tea that has numerous other health benefits like helping with colicky babies and soothing irritated skin. It is also delicious both "black" and with cream and sweetener.

Mint tea- while other scents can trigger hunger, peppermint suppresses your appetite. Try drink a cup of peppermint tea before main meals to benefit from this amazing effect.

Chapter 7: the one week tea cleanse plan for overall health and well being

Before you start your one-week plan, have a way to note exactly what you are drinking and how you feel as the plan progresses. This is going to help you identify the short term and long term effects of tea on your overall health. A journal or even a phone app would suffice.

Set your goals for the week. Do you just want a general detox to cleanse your system and assist with general well being or are you looking to lose weight? How you eat during your detox will also affect your outcome, regardless of your goal. Assist your body in feeling its best by nourishing it with healthy whole foods. As you are already planning to adopt new habits with tea this week, continue by having lots of fresh fruit, veggies, protein, and fibrous foods. This cleanse is not a "starve yourself" diet, but instead a plan to get in touch with what works best for your system to run optimally. Green tea and bacon double cheeseburgers with fries may not yield the results you desire...give your system a break by eating a well rounded diet and allowing your body to begin to heal itself.

During the detox program, aim to exercise for at least 20-30 minutes a day. Try vigorous exercise to increases your lymph flow and the circulation to help sweat out toxins. Vary with stretching such as yoga to open up body systems and deepen the detoxification process.

Drink plenty of water each day this week. This will also help to move the lymph and therefore assist the kidneys in detoxing, help flush fat, purify your body's cells, relieve constipation, stimulate the endocrine system, and rehydrate dry skin. Choose pure spring water. If you are not a big water drinker, try some fruit and vegetable smoothies. The smoothies have anti-oxidants that will help in detoxing and will also help in getting fluids into your body. Beware of sugar additives to your smoothies like juices or flavored yogurt. A little water and ice will help the smoothie blend nicely and add to your rehydration goals. Play around with flavors and mixtures. Hopefully you will find something you would like to keep in your routine!

Day 1: Getting Started

Today's focus is to get you used to drinking tea as a part of your daily routine. Let us keep it simple by using the detox green tea from Chapter 1. Happy sipping!

BREWING DETOX GREEN TEA

Yields: 1 serving

Ingredients

2 slices cucumber

2 strawberries sliced

1 teaspoon honey

1 slice lemon

1 green tea bag

Instructions

1.   Use the green tea bag and almost boiled water to brew 8-10 fluid ounces of green tea. Once the tea has steeped (3 minutes bagged or 4 minutes loose leaf), stir in the honey to dissolve.

2. Chill the green tea for 5 minutes in the refrigerator, remove, and add lemon, cucumber, and strawberries. Add ice if desired then stir to mix.

* Perhaps you could make a double batch to save you time throughout the day. Having a pitcher of tea readily available will help you to be more successful in accommodating this tea into your lifestyle. The longer the batch sets up in the refrigerator, the richer the flavors will become.

Day 2

This day, aim to take at least 2 cups of tea. Try the chai tea from Chapter 1. This tea will open your palate to a world of flavors and your system to amazing, healing spices to compliment the work of the tea. Today's tea is a hot tea. Note in your journal if you have any preference towards today tea over yesterday's iced version. Pay attention to how your body and mind are feeling. Also, remember to keep replacing processed foods in your menu with natural foods. It is pointless to help your body get rid of the toxins while you keep loading it with more. Help your body stay clean by eating clean food. Your system is doing hard work!

AYURVEDIC TEA, A DETOXING CHAI TEA

Ingredients

A squeeze of lemon

2 tablespoons green, black, or ginger tea

2 tablespoons fennel seeds

2 tablespoons cumin seeds

2 tablespoons coriander seeds

1 tablespoon thinly sliced fresh turmeric

2 tablespoons thinly sliced ginger

1 quart boiling water

Instructions

1.   Place all the ingredients in a French press and let it stand for 5 minutes before plunging and serving.

2.   Press can be refilled a second time using the ingredients for another infusion.

3. Alternatively, simmer all the ingredients together for 5 minutes in a pot and strain in a fine mesh strainer before drinking.

*The Golden Milk (Tumeric Milk) recipe from Chapter 1 would be a delicious addition to this flavorful tea!

Day 3

In addition, try to increase your tea intake to 3 cups. If you have preferred one of the teas from the previous days, make your life a little easier by repeating a familiar recipe. Also, venture out into a new tea experience. Perhaps, white tea for a lighter flavor would be a nice change of pace, particularly if you did not enjoy the rich flavor of yesterday's chai tea.

BREWING WHITE TEA

Yields: 1 serving

Ingredients

2 teaspoons white tea per cup

6 ounces of water

Instructions
5.   Bring water to a rolling boil then remove from heat.

6.   Add 2 teaspoons of white tea in the warm cup and fill the cup with very hot spring water.

Cover and steep for about 5 minutes.

*Try not adding sweetener to your white tea for one of your servings. Do you prefer it this way? If not, you can add a small amount of sweetener such as honey or even a low-glycemic teaspoon of coconut sugar and perhaps some milk of choice (dairy or nut/seed). Journal your preferences and how you are feeling today.

Day 4

Today will bring a new brain and heart healthy recipe. Not only are we going to experiment with a new ingredient, but also with a new way of making tea. Rosemary tea can help reduce stress and therefore drastically improve concentration. Studies have shown that rosemary counteracts the high levels of cholesterol in your blood through its phytochemicals, which naturally reduce LDL in the blood stream.

LEMON-ROSEMARY SUN TEA

Yields: 1 serving

Ingredients

1 ½ quarts cold water

¼ large lemon, thinly sliced

¼ cup fresh rosemary leaves (can be purchased in the produce section if you do not have fresh readily available to you)

Instructions

Bruise rosemary leaves with a wooden spoon in a large jar. Add the lemon and water, cover, and let this stand for 3-4 hours.

Strain and enjoy! Add a touch of sweetener and ice to serve immediately (or cool in the refrigerator). This tea can also be drunk in the morning to enjoy the benefits of mental clarity throughout your day.

*Please use a container that has been cleaned thoroughly with soap and water. Do not brew more tea than you will consume in that day and refrigerate it as soon as it's ready. Sun tea is a wonderful tradition in a lot of households, but safety should be at the forefront of your brewing. Please discard immediately if your tea has a stringy or ropey consistency. This is bacteria. Clean your vessel thoroughly before next use. If you enjoy the sun tea making process, it can be repeated with a variety of teas. Just add some bags to the water and steep per the instructions above. A little sweetener, lemons, ice, and a front porch will finish it nicely!

Day 5

Choose one of the teas from the previous days to accompany a healthy breakfast. The following tea should be drunk after lunch to help with digestive issues like heartburn and even bloating or gas. Drink this tea hot to help get things moving in your digestive system.

DIGESTIVE CHAI TEA RECIPE

Yields: 6 servings

Ingredients

2 tablespoons black tea

¾ teaspoon chopped licorice

1 tablespoon orange peel (organic orange preferred to avoid steeping chemicals)

2 tablespoons caraway seeds

2 tablespoons fennel seeds

2 tablespoons fenugreek seeds

8 cups water

Instructions

1.   Pour the water into a large pot and place the orange peel, seeds, licorice root into the water and cover. Simmer for 15 minutes, (much of the water will evaporate).

2.   Remove from the heat and add the black tea. Allow to steep while covered for 3 minutes. Strain and enjoy hot.

*Did you notice any digestive benefits from today's tea recipe? If so, write down your experiences. Your body has been on the detox journey for 5 days now. How are you enjoying the process? Stay positive! You only have a couple of more days in your one week plan.

Day 6

By now, you should be aiming for 5 cups of tea. We have tried a variety of recipes in the past 5 days. Return to a favorite or better yet, adventure into some of the other recipe suggestions you have seen in the book. Maybe through the detoxification process you have found your system fighting a cold. Try a fresh ginger tea of coined ginger boiled in water with a few peppercorns and honey. Maybe your digestive system is working hard and you are looking for a little relief. A cup of dandelion tea can help things move along while a cup of peppermint can sooth a variety of other stomach upsets. Maybe work is getting a little overwhelming and you need to focus on the big project coming up. Experiment with one of the teas in Chapter 5. You can always keep it simple by alternating a basic cup of green and black tea made to your preference. The point today is to be intentional about filling your system with delicious, healthful, antioxidant rich teas of your choosing. Make it a goal to have at least a cup with each meal and as a refreshing snack in the morning and afternoon. If time doesn't allow you to do so, that is ok. Double up a serving at breakfast or lunch!

*By now you certainly have preferences in your tea journey. What have been your favorites? Ones you could do without? Has your experience been work continuing as a part of your daily routine? Take a few moments as we look towards the last day to reflect. Have you noticed any changes in your body, your mind, your spirit?

Day 7

As you detox your body, it is also good to de-clutter your mind. Aim for at least 15 minutes of meditation on this particular day. You can start with the basics like belly breathing, i.e. if you don't know how to meditate. Start by placing your palm on your lower belly. Take a deep breath through the nose while counting slowly to 4. Feel your stomach rise when you breath in, then breathe out slowly and then let your belly to drop. Try to take this time while your tea is being prepared. Keep your meditation on things that create positivity in your life. Focus on memories, goals, or better yet, just being in the moment. This space is for you.

Continue with your 5 cups of tea today. Vary the cups or keep them consistent. Today is a day to reflect on what works best for you.

*Congratulations! You made it to the end of your one week tea cleanse! In addition to being mindful about drinking teas that are healing and restorative, you have been making great decisions for your body in terms of exercise and nutrition. Looking back, what are your thoughts? Finish up your journal entries today with an honest look at your experience this week. What have you learned? What will you hold onto? What will you let go?

Thank you for embarking on this journey. May health lead you forward as you continue to grow and learn more about your personal needs. Please join in one more chapter as we look at the benefits of tea not just for mind and body, but for your soul as well.

Chapter 8: the calm in the cup

Our lives are often planned, over-scheduled, and at times frantic. Cultivating a tea habit requires a small amount of time to slow down. Just the art of brewing a cup requires patience. Consider this, a hot cup of tea must be slowly sipped.

Sitting back and taking a tea break means reclaiming a moment in time for yourself. Imagine it as a mini-holiday. Protect that time. Often, it's stepping away from our stressors in life that gives us an opportunity for a new perspective, breakthrough, or idea. Little breaks in the long run can increase productivity, reduce anxiety, and make each of us a better employee, family member, and neighbor.

A cup of tea is also an excuse for you to get more liquids into your system. Dehydration when experiencing anxiety symptoms only makes the symptoms worse. Hydration helps our body systems function at a better rate. It helps to keep our bodies detoxification process in better shape. Aside from the numerous benefits mention above, the water in tea is an important bonus! When we have planned times to sit and enjoy a cup, we are assuring we are giving our systems the water that they need to best serve us and those we love.

To develop the habit of taking teas daily, you may want to anchor the new habit on something that you already do. If you read a newspaper or magazine daily, you can make an effort of taking tea each time you want to read. If you go for a run daily, you can take tea each time afterwards to rehydrate and to catch your breath. Anchoring the new habit of taking tea to an existing habit will help you continue this body, mind, and soul benefitting experience.

Take a tea break for you. Life is short though the days seem long. Plan to enjoy moments in each day before those moments are passed. Tea can be a healthy part of taking care of your whole person.

Chapter 9: what a tea cleanse is all about

For centuries, tea has been used as a natural remedy for common ailments. It is also an integral part of traditional healing methods. The healthy benefits obtained from various types of herbal teas cover practically everything. It can promote relief from the most common ailments like colds and indigestion to more serious ones like diabetes and cancer. Numerous studies over the years have found positive indications of the powerful effects of tea on health. Tea can lower risks for cardiovascular illnesses, reduce the threat of cancer, lower high blood pressure, improve lipid profile, enhance cognitive function and regulate mood. Tea can also help in achieving health goals such as stress relief and weight loss. Many studies into the efficacy of tea to promote various aspects of health have been performed and yielded favorable results. Teas can improve energy levels, enhance concentration, rev up metabolism, and help you in your weight loss goals.

Herbal teas are also effective in detoxifying the body. Herbal tea promotes cleansing through various steps. Different compounds promote toxin removal. They may act as magnets that draw out toxin buildup from within the cells while stimulating the liver to increase its detoxifying activities. Most teas have diuretic effects. This means that urination is promoted. This is another helpful step in cleansing the body. Toxins removed from within the tissues need to go somewhere and that's outside the body. Urination excretes a huge load of toxins and wastes from the body. Some teas promote superior digestion, which is another important factor that produces a wide scope of health benefits. One is that it promotes regular bowel movement. This will hasten the removal of wastes and toxins from the body.

While there are numerous supporting studies to the potency of tea, not all teas are the same. With the growing awareness on the health benefits of tea, a lot of companies are offering teas claimed to be effective. Not all teas are created equal. Some can work while others offer only false claims of improving health, promoting weight loss, or reducing stress. It is important that you learn what teas work for specific health goals and which ones do not.

How A Tea Cleanse Works

A tea cleanse is taking tea with the main goal of detoxifying the body. This is also called tea detox.

Most of the tea used for detox come with added ingredients. These added ingredients either enhance the tea's natural detox ability or function as the main detoxifying agent. Examples of commonly added ingredients are dandelion, ginger, lemon, and milk thistle. These ingredients support the liver's detoxification function. Ginger reduces oxidative stress on liver tissue, helping it to function optimally and still be healthy.

One ingredient to look out for when choosing tea for cleansing is senna. This is a fairly common ingredient that does help. It promotes the cleansing of the intestines, making the gut more effective at its digestive, absorptive, and excretory functions. Sennacontaining teas are taken at night. It is very effective, but only for short-term use. Prolonged use of senna can produce problems like dehydration, vomiting, electrolyte imbalances, and diarrhea. Daily cups of teas should be without any senna. Use only teas with senna for short-term tea cleanse.

A tea cleanse is very different from all other cleanse diets. You don't have to starve yourself. You eat normally and you still cleanse and lose weight. No starvation involved. All you have to do is choose among the recommended teas, eat the right kinds of food and enjoy the benefits.

Guidelines to Doing A 7 Day Tea Cleanse

By maintaining your tea cleanse for 7 consecutive days, you will promote more efficient excretion of the toxins within the cells and waste. While you can drink any time of the day, there are specific times when the most benefits can be obtained. If you aim to rev up your metabolism, drink tea upon waking up in the morning. It will jump-start your metabolism and keep it high throughout the day. If you want to de-stress or calm

146

down, take tea at bedtime. If you want to improve your digestion during a meal, take tea few minutes before eating. Then, work out a few more other cups throughout the day to keep the effects going.

Some people may be concerned over the amount of tea to be consumed in a day. When doing a tea cleanse, drink at least 5 to 7 cups of tea per day. This is perfectly fine. But, if sensitivity to caffeine is an issue, then decaffeinated versions should be used instead.

Combine your tea drinking with healthy eating as described in chapter 3 to ensure your body gets the most benefit out of your 7 day tea cleanse.

Chapter 10: best teas to start with

There are so many teas to choose from. There are natural herbal teas you can prepare for yourself. There are also commercially made, pre-mixed teas that promise cleansing and health. Not all of them are effective. Not all of them are great. Some teas are better than others for promoting particular health benefits.

The following are the top 5 Teas for health, whether you want to cleanse your body, boost metabolism, or achieve weight loss.

Green Tea

This is the leading tea for a variety of health benefits. It reduces cancer, treats certain cancers, promotes weight loss, improves brain function, detoxifies the body- and the list just goes on. More health benefits are being discovered about this wonderful tea as research progresses.

Green tea unlocks fat cells, making it easier for the body to burn them for energy. Drink green tea before a workout to boost the fat-blasting effect of your session. One study found that drinking 4-5 cups a day of green tea over a 7 day period, combined with a daily 25-minute workout session can promote the loss of up to an additional 10 pounds per week compared to those who did not drink green tea.

Catechins are responsible for most of green tea's benefits. They act as antioxidants that prevent free radical damage and reduce the effects of oxidative stress. These are also effective in collecting toxins from various tissues and bringing them to the blood. In turn, the blood can bring them to the liver for detoxification and to the gut and kidneys for excretion.

Oolong Tea

The name is a Chinese term that meant "black dragon". It is a light tea with floral notes. It is also full of catechins like green tea. This is better known as the tea that will make you lose 2 to 4 pounds in a week with daily use, even without exercise. This is accomplished by simply boosting the body's natural fat-burning process. Combined with exercise and an eating regime described later in this book, you can easily lose up to 10 pounds in a week.

Mint Tea

This is an effective appetite suppressing tea, without negative side effects. One cup of refreshing mint tea can suppress appetite for as long as 2 hours. Not only that, mint tea can promote better digestive process, helping you curb hunger and also get the most out of a meal. Most often, cravings for food are due to inadequate nutrients obtained from food because of poor digestion, meaning most of what you eat is partially digested and cannot be absorbed by the body. This will cause you to crave food that can provide quick energy, such as sugary food or refined carbs. To counter this, mint tea promotes more effective digestion of your meal, releasing the needed nutrients and energy your cells need. Your cells will no longer crave sugary, quick-energy food.

White Tea

This is an effective fat blocker that's great to add to your tea cleanse regimen. White tea prevents the formation of new fat cells, effectively inhibiting more fats to accumulate. This tea is made through natural drying processes, under the sun. This means white tea has undergone the least processing, compared to other kinds of teas. This preserves more of its compounds, making them intact and more useful. This is one reason why white tea contains up to 3 times more polyphenols than green tea.

One effect of white tea is boosting lipolysis and blocking adipogenesis. Lipolysis is the process that breaks down fat. Adipogenesis is the process that forms fat cells. White tea contains large concentrations of compounds that directly influence these processes, promoting weight loss and preventing fat formation. It is so potent that most experts consider white tea as a diet tea.

Rooibos Tea

This is the tea to help control your appetite. This is also an effective tea in regulating the hormones that influence fat storage. This tea comes from the leaves of a South African plant. This is the "red bush" plant, which exclusively grows in the small region of Cederberg, near Cape Town.

The most notable chemical in this tea is aspalathin. This is a potent flavonoid that can effectively reduce stress that stimulates hunger and accelerates fat storage.

Chapter 11: diet plan while on tea cleanse

The choice of tea for tea cleanse is important, as is the type of food you eat. You may be drinking the best tea for your cleansing and weight loss goals, but eating the wrong kind of food will hinder the success of your tea cleanse. Tea cleansing can only be effective if food is not taxing the rest of your system. You may be drinking the best tea available to clean your system but if you kept eating toxin-laden processed food, you still won't achieve the cleansing you desire. Tea won't be able to do much.

Choose your food properly, especially during a tea cleanse. This is vital to achieving a true cleanse. To help you make the best food choices, you have to carefully create a diet plan. You must be knowledgeable on food and its effects on the body.

Processed Food

This is the top food type to avoid. There is never anything good that can come out of processed food. The calories are empty and whatever "nutrient" present cannot be used effectively by the body. For example, processed food may contain carbohydrates, fats, and proteins. But the forms of these compounds are so heavily altered that they produce more harm than good in the body.

Processed food are full of artificial chemicals that become toxins in the body. Cutting out this type of food is doing a great service for your health. It will also allow the chosen tea to work to its full potential.

Learn to check your purchases. If the ingredient name is something you can't pronounce, there's a good chance you should avoid it. If something comes in a box, from a factory, it's probably been processed. The safest you can eat is fresh, whole, organically grown/raised food.

Refined Sugar and White Flour

These are among the worst foods for your body, and yet these ingredients are widely consumed as part of a standard western diet. Refined sugar and flour are present in so many foods, from processed food, baked goods, candies, even down to simple gravies and condiments. These have absolutely no nutritional value. White flour and sugar are involved in the development of insulin resistance, diabetes, obesity, and difficulty losing weight. During your tea cleanse you must avoid all food made with these at all cost.

Fried and Fatty Food

Fats are part of a balanced diet. But getting the unhealthy kind and in large amounts can produce negative effects in the body. Fried foods, for instance, contains so much fat. The kind of oil used for regular frying is also unhealthy. These can clog arteries. These are also quickly stored inside the tissues, seeing that the body has no use for it. Anything that the body cannot use are either stored of excreted. And because fats have the potential to be used as energy in the future, the body stores it. The problem is that a diet high in fat does not allow the body to use its fat stores. Instead, it promotes more storage.

Another problem arises when fat is oxidized in the body. It produces free radicals that destroy the integrity of the cell membrane. This triggers inflammation and more fat accumulation. It also increases the risk for cancers, cardiovascular diseases, stroke and obesity.

You can still incorporate fats in your diet. Just make sure it is from healthy sources and in controlled amounts. Good sources are plant oils like olive oil, coconut oil, flaxseed oil, and sesame oils. Fish oils are also great for health. These contain omega-3 fats that promote good health.

Avoid fried food, especially those from fast food such as french fries. Instead, choose healthier cooking methods such as broiling, steaming or baking. When using healthy fats, do so in moderation.

Fresh Vegetables

Fresh, whole, and organically grown vegetables should consist a major part of your daily diet. Macronutrients and micronutrients are abundant in vegetables. Green leafy vegetables are high in minerals and vitamins like vitamin B, magnesium, zinc and calcium. Brightly colored vegetables such as peppers and tomatoes are high in vitamins and minerals, along with antioxidants.

These antioxidants protect the cells from free radicals, remove free radicals, and excrete toxins from within the tissues.

Fresh Fruits

Fruits are also powerhouses for nutrients. But, be wise in choosing and eating fruits. There are some fruits that contain too much sugar. Some may contain smaller amounts but when eaten in large amounts, the sugar contents can add up.

Berries are the leading choice in healthy fruits. These are full of antioxidants that do your body good. Add berries to your tea cleanse diet plan and you are on your way to achieving good health in no time.

Whole Grains

These are healthy and rich sources of dietary fiber. This is vital in proper digestive function. Fiber acts as a mop that get wastes and toxins from the body, binding with them and then bringing them out to be excreted. This is an essential part of a tea cleanse because the toxins removed from the tissues need to be bound and excreted. Otherwise, it will just be recirculated.

Natural grains are way better than refined ones or those that come in cereal boxes. The less processing these grains underwent, the better they are. Try quinoa or brown rice instead of white rice.

Nuts, Beans, and Seeds

These are excellent sources of proteins. Eat these instead of animal proteins because they have less negative effects on the gut. Animal proteins tend to come with unhealthy fats, along with potential toxins from the antibiotics, artificial hormones, and commercial feeds they were raised with. If wanting to get animal proteins, choose those that were organically raised. Also, proteins from fishes are good alternatives, too.

Beans, seeds, and nuts are also high in fiber. Again, this is essential to successfully cleansing the body because it will promote excretion of unwanted chemicals, toxins, and wastes.

Chapter 12: teas that block fat

Certain teas contain specific compounds that effectively block fat. These compounds function in different ways, effecting different stages of the entire process of fat production, absorption, and accumulation.

From various researches, the top teas that block fat are the following:

White Tea

White tea contains natural compounds that shuttle or remove fat from the body. This is also the richest source of antioxidant in the world of tea. The polyphenols found in white tea is 3 times more than the amount found in green tea. The best white tea is naturally dried, especially those dried under natural sunlight.

Compounds in white tea work double. These simultaneously block off fat cell formation while boosting breakdown of fat.

The antioxidants in white tea also helps in fighting off fats. These compounds stimulate cells to release their fat contents. Then these antioxidants will trigger the liver to speed up its fat-burning processes. This process will convert fats released from within the cells into usable energy.

Green Tea

This tea acts on the genes that regulate fat. Green tea influences these genes and reverses the fat-storing effects. The catechin EGCG can be found in large amounts in green tea. This EGCG affects genetic triggers for obesity and diabetes. By turning off the involved genes, EGCG risk for diabetes and obesity are greatly reduced. Not only that, EGCG boosts CCK levels. CCK is a hormone that has hunger-suppressing effects in the body.

Black Tea

This is another great tea that helps in fighting fat. It lowers the levels of hormones that promote fat storage. Brew and enjoy black tea the next time you are stressed out. It also fights the negative effects of stress and helps you relax.

According to studies, stress increases the level of the hormone adrenaline. This hormone is involved in the body's fight-or-flight response. It also affects fat metabolism and regulation. In the presence of adrenaline, the fat cells are stimulated to release fatty acids. These fatty acids can be used by the various tissues as energy needed for the fight-or-flight response. However, in chronic stress, adrenaline levels remain high for an extended period. The result is that too many fatty acids are released into the blood. The excess fatty acids are then converted into fatty deposits.

Another hormone affected by high stress levels is cortisol. This hormone has direct influence over fat and fat storage. Cortisol converts fatty acids in the blood into fat cells. Then, these fat cells are brought to the belly area where they will be stored. Fat stored in the belly is the most difficult to burn. This belly fat also has more serious effects on health compared to other stored fats. It contributes to hormonal imbalances that promote more fat storage. It is also involved in the development of health problems like obesity, diabetes and cardiovascular issues.

Black tea quickly reduces the levels of adrenaline and cortisol in the body. It provides relaxation and brings down stress hormone levels quickly. This will limit the fat-promoting effects of adrenaline and cortisol. The relaxing effect will block fat production and accumulation.

Barberry Tea

Barberry tea is effective in limiting growth of cells. It prevents the fat cells from further growth and from becoming larger. The most notable compound in barberry tea is berberine. This chemical occurs naturally and is found in the barberry shrub. This chemical is effective in preventing weight gain. This effect can still be seen even when eating a diet high in fat. This compound is also effective in protecting the cells from insulin resistance.

When drinking barberry tea, energy expenditure is enhanced. The surface receptors on fat cells are also decreased. This will make them less receptive and responsive to incoming fat sources.

Rooibos Tea

This tea has the ability to inhibit fat cell formation. Studies have found that the flavonoids and the polyphenols in rooibos tea stop fat cell formation by 22%.

The flavonoid aspalathin is a particularly potent chemical in rooibos tea. This chemical is effective for the reduction of stress hormones involved in hunger cues and storage of fats.

Pu-erh Tea

This tea is effective in shrinking or reducing the size of the fat cells. Pu-erh tea is made from fermented tea. This is effective in lowering the concentrations of triglycerides in the body. This is a type of fat that can be potentially dangerous in large concentrations. Also, pu-erh tea reduces fat accumulated around the belly area. This tea is especially helpful for those who consume a high fat diet.

Chapter 13: teas that boost metabolism

Green Tea

Among the long list of green tea's benefits is fat reduction. The compounds in green tea promote the conversion of fat into readily usable energy. Just 1 cup of green tea can already do wonders to your metabolism, cranking it up, and boosting energy.

One recent study found that people can experience fat loss in the belly area with green tea. Regularly drinking 4 to 5 cups daily can help in losing up to 10 pounds of predominantly belly fat per week on average. Drinking green tea daily should be combined with at least 25 minutes of exercise.

The catechins are responsible for this effect. This is a kind of antioxidant in green tea that acts on fat cells.

These chemicals trigger fat release from fat cells and then boost the liver's fat-transformation processes. This will produce more energy for the body to use and reduce fat stores.

Oolong Tea

This tea can help you burn about 1 pound a week. This is a traditional Chinese tea that is particularly rich in antioxidants. Cholesterol levels are effectively controlled by the compounds in oolong tea. Digestion is also improved. Not only that, oolong tea effectively revs up the body's metabolic rate.

The abundance of catechins in this tea is responsible for the metabolism-boosting action. This supports weight loss because it promotes fat metabolism.

Yerba maté Tea

This tea enhances the positive effects of your workout. The thermogenic effect of yerba maté is its leading benefit. This effect is turning up the body's ability to burn calories. Thermogenic effect means this tea increases the body's calorie burning process.

Aside from speeding up the calorie burning process, yerba maté promotes weight loss by influencing insulin activity. The compounds in yerba maté improves insulin sensitivity.

One study found that yerba maté tea enhances the benefits of a workout. People who consumed the tea had higher levels of metabolic improvements compared to those working out without taking the tea.

Goji Tea

This tea showed positive effects on calorie burning. It has been found that it can increase calorie burning by as much as 10%.

Goji berries are becoming more and more popular for their health benefits. Taking them as tea can also have positive effects on metabolism. The plant, Lycium barbarum, is the source of the popular goji berries. This plant is part of the traditional medicinal therapy in Asian healing practices. This is used for the treatment of several ailments such as diabetes. Taken as tea, goji can also provide dramatic slimming results. One study found that those who took goji tea experienced a 10%

boost in their metabolism compared to those who did not. This effect was observed during a study where participants took goji after a meal. The enhanced caloric burning lasted for 4 hours.

Kola Nut Tea

The tea from kola nut is also effective in boosting metabolism. Often, just a single cup daily is enough to achieve this benefit.

Chapter 14: teas that flatten the tummy

Teas can help you get a flat stomach. One way this occurs is by promoting better digestion. If food is digested fully, you get more nutrients and less waste. Your tissues function better too because they get good quality fuel to work with. That means less "sludge" that can promote fat formation and accumulation.

Bloating is the accumulation of gas and undigested materials within the gut. This is often caused by poor peristalsis or movement of the digestive tract. This contributes to making the belly area look bigger than it really is. By reducing bloating, your tummy will surely look flatter even without much exercise. Teas also lessen bloating, helping to further flatten the belly area.

The best teas for promoting improved digestion and reducing bloating include:

Green Tea

It would be more surprising if green tea is not included in any list of natural remedies and health-promoting activities. Green tea helps clean the body and get rid of toxins. It also promotes better digestion. Recent studies discovered that green tea also helps with weight loss. Compounds in this healthy tea speeds up the body's metabolic rate and rate of fat burning. These will contribute to flattening the stomach. Daily consumption of at least 3 cups unsweetened green tea will give this benefit.

Catechins in green tea is found to increase the activity of pepsin. This is a digestive enzyme responsible for breaking down proteins. Undigested and partially digested proteins contribute to bloating. Green tea helps the stomach to fully digest these particles and prevent bloating.

Peppermint Tea

This is commonly used as a natural digestive aid. Peppermint tea can also reduce bloating by stimulating regular, normal rhythmic movement of the gut. Take peppermint tea after each meal to promote better digestive rhythm and reduce bloating. Organic and unsweetened peppermint tea is more effective for this purpose compared to the sweetened variety.

Peppermint tea also stimulates the gall bladder. It triggers the release of more bile, improving its flow into the gut. Bile is vital for fat digestion. In adequate amounts, bile binds with fat, making it easier for the other digestive enzymes to act on the fat molecules. This promotes quicker fat digestion, which effectively reduces bloating.

This tea is not for everyone, though. Those taking diabetic medications, suffering from high blood pressure and acid reflux should avoid peppermint tea.

Ginger Tea

This is another popular herb to aid digestion. Ginger compounds also detoxify the blood, removing toxins and reducing the incidence of bloating. The best results are achieved by drinking a cup of tea from a fresh root. Take a fresh ginger root, wash it well and slice into smaller pieces. Boil water and add the sliced roots. Boil the root for 10 minutes. Strain and drink as it is, without adding sweeteners. Drink 3 times a day, preferably after every meal.

Caution is advised with taking ginger tea for certain conditions. Those suffering from high blood pressure, taking diabetic medications, and those on blood-thinner medications should avoid ginger tea.

Lemon Tea

This is a great cleansing tea that can effectively reduce bloating. Lemon tea effectively flattens the stomach with daily intake. It is also very easy to make. Pour boiling hot water in a cup and then squeeze 1 whole lemon into it. Mix and drink unsweetened for maximum results. Adding organic honey is also good because honey also supports the digestive tract. Drink 3 times a day before a meal to promote better appetite control. Drink after meals to promote better digestion.

Chai Tea

This tea is made by combining different spices such as ginger, pepper, cinnamon and cardamom. These spices are responsible for the belly flattening effect of chai tea. For instance, cinnamon relieves digestive ailments like indigestion, gas, nausea, stomach cramps and heartburn. Ginger improves digestive processes, relieving nausea and upset stomach.

Chamomile Tea

Gas and indigestion can be relieved with chamomile tea. It can also be used to relieve constipation. If bowel movements are not regular, then toxins and other wastes will stay longer in the large intestines. The longer they stay there, the bad bacteria in the gut will feed on the wastes and the by-product of this will be gas and bloating. This will also promote gut imbalance that can contribute to poor digestion, bloating, and more fat accumulation. Take chamomile tea to promote regular bowel movement.

Chamomile is also effective in providing relief from cramps and other problems in the gut. The compounds in chamomile have a gentle sedative effect that quiet down inflammation in the lining of the gut. This effect also reduces heartburn and flatulence.

Chamomile is effective but is not recommended for everyone. Those who have allergies to ragweed or those who find themselves sneezing when exposed to asters or chrysanthemum should not take chamomile. Allergic symptoms and sensitivity reactions may worsen with chamomile.

Lemon Balm Tea

This herb is in the same family as other minty herbs like peppermint and spearmint. It can relieve pains from gas as well as bloating resulting from indigestion. The most notable chemicals in lemon balm that produce its health benefits are eugenol and the terpenes.

Chapter 15: tea to relieve stress

Stress causes the release of both adrenaline and cortisol. This tandem will promote greater fat production and accumulation. Adrenaline promotes fatty acids to be released from the fat cells. Then, cortisol will act on these fatty acids and convert them to fat. This is the reason why most people with chronically high levels of stress often have large belly fat.

Aside from the direct effects of these two stress hormones, there is another side effect. Stress puts the body on higher alert. That means the cells are needing more energy than usual. But because fatty acids meant for energy use are quickly converted into fats and then stored, an energy deficit is created. The cells do not get the energy they need. These cells will send a signal to the body seek additional calories. Notice when you are stressed out, you crave foods that are high in calories and sugar. That is your cells signaling for quick energy.

Tea can help reduce stress. Most often, teas come in pre-packed tea bags ready to be steeped. Just place one bag in a cup of hot water and steep for 5 minutes. The longer tea is steeped, the more concentrated it becomes.

The best teas to use for stress relief are:

Mint Tea

Spearmint and peppermint have a refreshing aroma. They help relax the mind and reduce anxiety.

Chamomile Tea

Chamomile has a soothing effect on the nerves. It promotes calmness both of the mind and the body. Hyperactive people will find drinking chamomile tea helpful. It can help in stabilizing their moods. Those who have difficulty sleeping may also find themselves sleeping sooner and better after drinking chamomile tea.

Ginseng

This is among the most popular and oldest herb used for healing and promoting better health. Ginseng helps in clearing out mental exhaustion. It also helps in easing away stress. After a cup of soothing ginseng tea, you will feel calmer and more peaceful. Also, ginseng can help improve sleep.

Skullcap

This can help ease tension from the muscles. Drinking skullcap can also help in reducing muscle spasms and headaches. It is also effective in calming the nerves. Women experiencing premenstrual syndrome may also experience less irritability.

Lavender Tea

Tension headaches are a frequent occurrence among the population. This is brought about by stress. Lavender tea is an effective measure to promote relief. It relieves exhaustion of the nervous system. It also helps resolve problems with indigestion. The relief helps reduce cortisol and adrenaline levels that can help with weight loss and health.

Linden Tea

This promotes relaxation of both nerves and muscles. It calms the mind and relieves stress-related headaches.

Valerian Tea

This is a popular herbal tea, best known for the sedative properties. Valerian tea is a common natural remedy for those who have trouble falling sleep. It can also ease tension, whether it's emotional stress or a physical discomfort. Exercise caution in taking valerian tea. Drinking too much can cause lethargy. Also, this is not advisable for children younger than 12 years old.

Lemon Balm Tea

Lemon balm is effective in soothing the body and calming the mind. Its soothing effect is directed at the nervous system. It promotes reduction of nervousness making you feel less upset or anxious. Steep lemon balm for 15 minutes and drink as hot tea or iced tea.

Kava Tea

A cup of kava tea can treat moderate to severe anxiety. It can reduce the incidence of thoughts that promote anxiety. Kava is very effective but there are some concerns over its use, especially among those with chronic health issues and taking certain medications. It is best to consult a doctor first before taking kava.

Hops

Hops is a main ingredient in brewing beer. But this can also be made into tea. Hops tea can reduce stress and nervousness. Hops can also help a weakened immune system due to stress.

Green Tea

Of course, green tea includes stress relief in its long list of benefits. The amino acid theanine promotes relaxation in the body. Studies found that this amino acid affects the brain's alpha waves. This is involved in the process of promoting relaxation. However, it is more advisable to take the decaffeinated version because the caffeine content can counter the calming effect.

CALENDULA TEA

Also referred to as pot marigold, Calendula is an aromatic plant that can be easily grown in the garden. It is native to Southern Europe. For many years, it has been used as an herbal medicine for the treatment of fever, inflammation, and wounds, among others. Its pungent odor also makes it effective as an insect repellant.

Why Calendula Tea is good for you

Calendula is believed to aid in digestive function. It works effectively in treating gastric ulcers and digestive inflammation. It's not only anti-inflammatory; it also possesses anti-viral and anti-fungal properties.

This tea is also excellent for detoxification. It induces urine production and encourages the elimination of toxic wastes from the body. Overall, Calendula can help prevent and treat diseases and at the same time, strengthen immunity.

How to make Calendula Tea

This basic Calendula Tea recipe makes two servings.

Ingredients:

-2 teaspoons of dried Calendula florets

-2 cups of water

Directions:

1.Boil water with dried Calendula florets in a kettle over medium heat.

2.Once boiling, remove from heat and allow it to steep for 10 or up to 15 minutes.

3.Strain the infusion and serve.

*You can have 3 cups of this concoction a day. If the taste is too strong, you may add 1 teaspoon of honey for every cup of Calendula tea.

Additional Tips and Reminders in Making Calendula Tea
Calendula can be easily grown in your own backyard. You can make tea using the fresh flowers. Alternatively, you can dry them first before making an infusion. You may use 1 teaspoon of dried Calendula florets to make a cup of tea. If you're using fresh florets, 2 teaspoons should be mixed for every cup of water. Calendula is also available in health food stores in the form of herbal tea bags.

Side Effects and Precautions
It is generally safe for adults to consume Calendula Tea and there are no side effects reported regarding its use. However, sensitive people may experience symptoms of allergic reactions. If such occurs, you should stop using the tea immediately. People who are allergic to either ragweed or daisy are likely allergic to Calendula as well.

APPLE CIDER TEA

Seriously, is there anything that Apple Cider Vinegar can't fix? It is literally an age-old wonder. You can drink it or use it as a cooking ingredient to reap the healthy benefits.

Why Apple Cider Tea is good for you

Among the most important benefits of apple cider vinegar is its malic acid content which works effectively in clearing clogged lymph nodes, arteries and organ tissues, thereby improving heart health. When applied topically, apple cider can also promote skin health. In fact, it is an effective treatment for acne, skin discolorations, warts and blemishes. It is also an excellent remedy for insomnia and heartburn. In addition, it can help with weight loss.

A research study published in the Bioscience, Biotechnology and Biochemistry journal in 2009 reported that 3 months of drinking apple cider vinegar could lead to significant weight loss specifically in the reduction of waist circumference and abdominal fat. You can improve digestion and energy levels with this tea recipe. The addition of lemon juice further boosts its weight loss and detox properties.

HOW TO MAKE APPLE CIDER TEA

Because drinking apple cider vinegar on its own may prove challenging to wash down and can possibly destroy tooth enamel, drink this recipe to overcome the challenges. It makes one serving.

Ingredients:

-1 cup of hot water

-1 teaspoon of freshly squeezed lemon juice

-1 teaspoon of honey

-1 tablespoon of apple cider vinegar

Directions:

1.Heat water to boiling point. Set it aside for 3 minutes to cool.

2.Pour the hot water into a cup. Next, add the apple cider vinegar and honey. Stir it well.

3.Stir in the freshly squeezed lemon juice and enjoy!

Additional Tips and Reminders in Making Apple Cider Tea

This Apple Cider Vinegar tea is best consumed before each meal. It can help you curb your appetite. If you're not comfortable taking it on an empty stomach, you can also enjoy it after each meal to control your cravings. You can have the tea 2 or 3 times each day. Skip the honey in this recipe if you prefer, but it really enhances the apple flavor of the tea.

Side Effects and Precautions

There is no danger in consuming apple cider vinegar. However, you should limit your consumption to 3 tablespoons a day. It is also not advisable for you to drink it on its own. You should always dilute it with water or mix it up. That is why this apple cider tea recipe is just perfect!

AYURVEDA DETOX TEA

Ayurvedic teas are known for their soothing properties and ability to treat various ailments. With the right ingredients, you can also use them to boost weight loss. That's exactly what this Ayurvedic tea does. It combines coriander, fennel seeds and cumin to create a powerful detox drink to help you kiss belly flat goodbye!

Why Ayurveda Detox Tea is good for you

Coriander is native to West Asia, North Africa and South Europe. It's known to provide flavor for stir-fries, snacks, curries, salsa, meat dishes and burritos. While the leaves are commonly used for cooking, the seeds make a great tea for promoting beautiful skin and hair growth. Coriander tea can also help treat diabetes and the common cold or flu. In addition, coriander helps improve digestion.

Coriander's rich source of dietary fiber and antioxidants work well in facilitating bowel movements and keeping the liver healthy. It also contains digestive juices and compounds that promote better digestion.

What Fennel seeds bring to the table is dietary fiber, lots of it! You are probably aware of the crucial role that fiber plays in the weight loss game. It not only gives you the feeling of fullness, but also encourages bowel movements and toxin elimination.

Cumin, fennel and coriander seeds are all spices. That means they help in increasing metabolic rate and fat burning. You can use them separately or all together like in the following recipe.

How to make Ayurveda Detox Tea

With small amounts of cumin, fennel and coriander seeds, this tea recipe is an amazing detox drink. This recipe makes one serving.

Ingredients:

-1 1/2 cups of water

-1/4 teaspoon of fennel seeds

-1/4 teaspoon of coriander seeds

-1/4 teaspoon of cumin

Directions:

1.Boil water in a kettle over medium high heat.

2.Once boiling, add the cumin, fennel and coriander seeds.

3.Reduce heat to simmer for 5 minutes.

4.Strain the mixture and serve.

Additional Tips and Reminders in Making Ayurveda Detox Tea

Coriander is very flavorful and fennel has a mild licorice taste. If the taste of this tea is too strong for you, you can either try one seed at a time or cut the portions in half and work your way up until you get used to it.

Side Effects and Precautions

The recommended dosage is 3 cups a day. Although there are no known side effects for this natural remedy, it is best to practice caution. If you are suffering from a medical condition, it would be wise to consult with your doctor first. In addition, pregnant women are advised against taking this weight loss remedy. Sensitive people may develop allergic reactions so watch out for symptoms.

Conclusion

Thank you again for downloading this book!

I hope this book was able to help you to learn how to cleanse with tea. More than that, I hope this book helped you to put into perspective habits and routines that allow you to live your most healthy and energized life.

Revisit the one week cleanse as needed. Otherwise, keep enjoying your mini-holiday one cup at a time!

Thank you and best wishes for a healthier you!

www.ingramcontent.com/pod-product-compliance
Lightning Source LLC
Chambersburg PA
CBHW062135020426

42335CB00013B/1228